BEST PRACTICES I
The Classroom As An Assessment Arena

Katharine G. Butler, PhD
Editor, *Topics in Language Disorders*
Syracuse University
Syracuse, New York

TOPICS IN LANGUAGE DISORDERS SERIES

AN ASPEN PUBLICATION®
Aspen Publishers, Inc.
Gaithersburg, Maryland
1994

Library of Congress Cataloging-in-Publication Data

Best practices / Katharine G. Butler, editor.
p. cm.
Compilations from: Topics in language disorders.
Includes bibliographical references and index.
Contents: 1. The classroom as an assessment arena—2. The
classroom as an intervention context.
ISBN: 0-8342-0586-6 (v. 1)—ISBN: 0-8342-0587-4 (v. 2)
1. Handicapped children—Education—Language arts. 2. Language
disorders in children—Treatment 3. Speech therapy for children.
4. Speech disorders in children—Diagnosis.
5. Learning disabled children—Education—Language arts.
I. Butler, Katharine G. II. Topics in language disorders
LC4028.B47 1994
371.91'4—dc20
93-36264
CIP

Editorial Resources: Ruth Bloom

Library of Congress Catalog Card Number: 93-36264
ISBN: 0-8342-0586-6
Series ISBN: 0-8342-0590-4

Printed in the United States

1 2 3 4 5

Table of Contents

Best Practices I: The Classroom As an Assessment Arena

Preface

Topics in Language Disorders is a transdisciplinary journal that is devoted to discussion of issues surrounding language acquisition and its disorders. *TLD* has as its major purposes (1) providing relevant information to practicing professionals who provide services to those who are at-risk or have language disabilities; (2) clarifying the application of theory and research to practice; (3) bringing together professionals across disciplines, who are researchers and clinicians from the health and education arenas both as authors and as readers; (4) clarifying the application of theory to practice among professionals and students-in-training; and (5) contributing to the scientific literature while making each issue accessible and relevant to an interdisciplinary readership.

Typically, each *TLD* journal is devoted to single topic, although the constellation of articles may vary. A few may be wholly clinical in nature, while most blend practice and research. In the *TLD* book series, each book provides a critical but highly sensitive evaluation of current research and translates that analysis into a framework for service delivery. Hence, in this *TLD* book, the reader will find a distillation of the best of the journal's current offerings as well as some seminal articles that may enhance readers' conceptual knowledge. Offerings are provided by professionals from a variety of disciplines: speech-language pathology, psychology, reading, learning disabilities, curriculum and instruction, speech communication, language education, English, writing, regular and special education. This text focuses on the classroom as a context for assessment, highlighting proven as well as experimental procedures and possibilities.

PART I. LOOKING AT CHILDREN IN THE SCHOOLS: SOME CLASSROOM INSIGHTS

As the nation's schools have become more culturally and ethnically diverse, all professionals who work with students are being required to develop new skills. Time-honored approaches in assessment and intervention have been found wanting in the American schools of today and tomorrow. For example, of every 100 children enrolled in California public schools in the Fall of 1993, 17 live below the poverty level, 21 are Limited-English-Proficient (LEP) and 7 live in abusive family situations. Enrollment currently stands at 5.7 million, and the general consensus is that approximately half of that number are increasingly troubled (McCormick, 1993). Changes in children are accompanied by changes in educational approaches to resolve school-based language and learning difficulties. The emphasis has shifted from standardized assessment instruments to authentic tasks requiring authentic communication in authentic contexts of home or school. The problem, of course, is that home and school are each "authentic" in its own way, and that the authenticity of one's own culture may not be replicated in another's. Thus, it is that language specialists have adopted or adapted some of anthropology's approaches to studying the cultures of others. Specifically, ethnography has "a long history of use in understanding communication patterns within diverse cultures" and of assisting language specialists "in understanding variations in communicative interactions and the rules for these variations" (Westby & Erickson, 1992, p. vii).

Therefore, Part I begins with García's enlightening article on "Ethnography and Classroom Communication: Taking an Emic Perspective." García draws upon the research of sociolinguists and classroom ethnographers who study the role of language in school instruction and of educational anthropologists who view the language of the home, community, and school within a cultural context. Assessing children's communicative competence in the classroom and their response to the demands of the teacher, García maintains that even in whole language classrooms most teachers remain as authority figures. As a result children must comprehend and use the most common patterns of classroom interaction known as IRE (The teacher Initiates a question, the student Responds, and the teacher Evaluates.). Readers will find a number of home-school discontinuities elaborated by García based upon research conducted via extensive participant observations and detailed analyses of video- or tape-recorded speech events. As García concludes, "a key component of the emic perspective is the ability to observe others from their perspective and to understanding how one is conditioned by one's own perspective." Necessary prerequisites are the ability to observe that which has been unobserved, search for alternative explanations for the unexplained, and to step outside one's own culture.

Over the past decade, language specialists, reading teachers, and learning disabilities teachers have debated the merits of "whole language." Sawyer, in "Whole Language in Context: Insights into the Current Great Debate," provides information on reading instruction—past, present, and future. In so doing, she also presents the whole language view of literacy acquisition and how literate behavior is promoted in this setting. She asserts that "code emphasis programs and the bottom-up approach in general is eroding." Her evaluation concludes with the observation that learning disabled children who require direct teaching may be well served if this occurs in a whole language classroom.

Nelson, in "Individual Processing in Classroom Settings," returns to the ecological motif, and adds that system theory is also very helpful for looking at how individual children process classroom information. She also cites five pragmatic indicators for identifying children at risk for language disabilities: they include: (1) nonfluent self-expression, (2) unusual delays before responding, (3) nonexplicit and ambiguous vocabulary use, (4) irrelevant responses, and (5) poor topic maintenance. Nelson's

comments span the assessment arena's requirements: parental interview and history-taking, interviews with teachers, student interviews, direct and indirect observation of the student's classroom interactions and a review of curricular material. Over time, Nelson has fine-tuned her curriculum-based assessment procedures. Her work has become increasingly important, not only in the assessment sphere, but also through intervention procedures that are derived from a systems approach. Nelson closes with a sage remark: she encourages assessors to partition a problem "so that it becomes more manageable without losing sight of the system as a whole."

"Questions: A Powerful but Misused Form of Classroom Exchange" by Blank and White is a seminal article that introduced many readers to the IRE mode of teacher-student exchanges. As Blank and White note, classroom exchanges are frequently unlike any question-answer procedure encountered elsewhere. Classroom dialogue is a unique attribute of the school, one that is taken for granted within that setting by adults present, but may contribute to children's difficulties who have neither experienced it elsewhere or whose cultural and linguistic perspective differs. The authors provide suggestions for using questions to create a shared context and using questions to avoid explicit criticism. They conclude: "Questions need not be abandoned; rather their misuse should be curbed so that constructive uses can emerge."

In the final article in Part I, Rubin, a well-known language educator, defines those areas that contribute to the "Divergence and Convergence between Oral and Written Communication." Rubin turns to the subject of Black English Vernacular (BEV) speakers and how they write. He maintains that "no one is a native speaker of writing, not SE (Standard English) speakers and not BEV speakers. All novice writers must learn to switch into the written code, and nonstandard-dialect speakers are about as successful (or unsuccessful) as any other." He concludes that spoken and written styles diverge in many ways, but also converge in certain respects. He concludes with a reprise of how structured oral communication experiences can provide grist for the composing mill process as well as providing for what he terms as "cognitive calisthenics" for developing skills that underlie writing ability. Readers will find his suggestions illuminating.

PART II. LANGUAGE ASSESSMENT AND LITERACY DEVELOPMENT

Returning to the ethnographic perspective cited in Part I, Fishman provides further evidence in "Ethnography and Literacy: Learning in Context." She provides two exemplars, one of Daniel, who attends a school in an Old Order Amish community. The second is Mitch, a student in a residential school for juvenile delinquents. One of the author's most interesting comments is a reflection on teachers and their interest in their students' written products. Fishman points out that these two students differ in many ways, but that both "do as much as necessary to meet assignment requirements and as little as they can to achieve the same ends...these students 'read' their assignments, their teachers, and their cultures perfectly. They know what is actually required and what really is not necessary or valued." She notes that both of these students ask, "What's in it for me?" What's more, she answers that (and other) questions to the readers' satisfaction.

Unknown to speech-language pathologists a few decades ago, script reports have become part of the vernacular. As Ross and Berg point out in "Individual Differences in Script Reports: Implications for Language Assessment," a script "has been defined as a set of expectations individuals have about routine events that is organized in a temporal-casual sequence of acts or single actions." The task the

authors set for themselves is to provide readers some idea of how individual differences in scripts may produce idiosyncratic verbal reports that are not necessarily deviant, but rather, reflect the child's memory of previous experiences. These results are discussed in terms of both tests assessing language comprehension that involve memory for events and also elicited language samples that tap into recall of past events. A portion of the message for readers conveys the notion that a "routine" event in one child's life may be anything but routine in another's. The authors conclude that clinicians should be careful in drawing conclusions from script reports since "differential experiences...may result in impoverished or elaborate scripts."

Silliman, Wilkinson, and Hoffman provide a cutting-edge description of "Progress in Language and Literacy Learning: Ongoing Assessment in the Classroom." These authors have done a remarkable job of conveying to readers what it really means to convert a philosophy of language, its acquisition, and use in classroom settings to a framework for truly authentic assessment. Many use such words, but few complete the microanalyses that actualizes the assessment construct. In a tour de force, the authors review the types of observational tools used in the assessment of authentic progress and then describe in detail their use (narrative tools, portfolio collections, running records, critical incidents, and descriptive tools) and the outcomes of their use. This truly collaborative enterprise can serve as a model for school systems large or small whose language professionals wish to accomplish similar goals. Readers will also enjoy the commentary that provides the concluding section of this discussion. The authors identify their successes by discussing the benefits of the program—its "intended effects." They also specify, as do all good researchers, the "unintended effects." Readers will enjoy and benefit from both.

Creaghead provides an illuminating and seminal article in "Comprehension of Meaning in Written Language," as she explores the role of the oral language specialist on the "reading team," a controversial statement in the 1980s, and perhaps, alas, in the 1990s. Creaghead comments on author and audience considerations, on taking the perspective of the listener/reader, on the importance of scripts, and of using context to predict meaning. She concludes that an integrated experience approach to reading is most helpful, and she cites the language specialist as a uniquely qualified individual to assist language-impaired children in this endeavor.

Catts continues the theme in his article addressing "Early Identification of Reading Disabilities." He reminds readers that there is life before kindergarten and early reading instruction. Improving early identification of reading difficulties requires that professionals carefully look at the preschool years in a more comprehensive manner. Catts traces the history of language and reading disabilities, phonological awareness deficits, word retrieval problems, and verbal memory deficits. He concludes that early reading problems may well be rooted in the oral language problems of the preschool years. While calling for future research initiatives, he amply illustrates the need for language specialists and reading specialists to work together in early identification and assessment.

Carlisle supports Nelson's earlier commentary by specifying that professionals move beyond norm-referenced tests in "Planning an Assessment of Listening and Reading Comprehension." She stresses the importance of what can be learned about comprehension problems by assessment of discourse through listening and reading. Following a brief review of the developmental aspects of the relationship between listening and reading, she moves directly to the problems associated with selecting text passages and methods of testing

comprehension. She provides a protocol for designing a test to compare listening and reading, and provides an exemplar and two case studies. In conclusion, Carlisle provides a convincing argument that evaluation of extended discourse is an essential procedure in the identification of reading difficulties.

Snyder and Godley, in "Assessment of Word-Finding Disorders in Children and Adolescents," provide a view of children's word-finding problems commenting on the fact that "words are the very 'stuff' of which language is made." Assessment should include a systematic approach to the measurement of naming and word retrieval. Screening for word-finding difficulties in the classroom is possible via teacher referral as well as by clinician observation in the classroom setting. Direct assessment should follow, and Snyder and Godley provide the prerequisite activities and the types of instruments that can be used. A comprehensive assessment is highly recommended, and instruments used therein are critiqued. Experienced clinicians will celebrate the authors' concluding statements: "One would think that naming objects, actions, and conditions is a relatively simple and straightforward process and that the assessment of this verbal skill would be similarly direct. The complexity of language production, however, is such that even a task so apparently simple as naming can be influenced by many factors...." Readers are encouraged to consult the article for final statements.

For those who wonder if and when computerized language sampling will be an every-day accoutrement in the schools, Miller, Frieberg, Rolland, and Reeves have the answer in "Implementing Computerized Language Sample Analysis in the Public School." More than 60 speech-language pathologists working in the public schools have participated in the project reported in the article. Using both conversation and narratives, examiners collected the language samples required for the data base. The need for SLPs who are mentors to others in their school districts is noted, as well as the use of nonprofessionals to transcribe the language samples. The authors discuss the pros and cons of the latter activity as well as the diversity of language disorders as seen from the perspective of this large data base. They conclude that language sampling is crucial for identifying and describing language disorders. Finally, the authors note that portable computers would do much to ease the SLPs' responsibilities in the identification and monitoring of intervention services.

If the classroom is the appropriate setting for assessment of language disorders for mild to moderately language impaired, what of the more difficult and/or more severely disabled? This issue is addressed in Part III.

PART III. LANGUAGE ASSESSMENT OF SOME OF THE MORE SEVERELY LANGUAGE IMPAIRED

Classroom teachers and parents must be more involved in language assessment of their charges. Light and McNaughton address this issue in "Literacy and Augmentative and Alternative Communication (ACC): The Expectations and Priorities of Parents and Teachers." Similarities and differences between parents and teachers were explored by the authors and the results reported. Priorities are likewise addressed. The authors acknowledge that research on expectations and priorities is limited. The need for greater knowledge is obvious. Appropriate assessment leads to more effective instruction—the authors stress the importance of garnering this knowledge.

Blosser and DePompei provide the final comment, as they discuss "The Head-Injured Student Returns to School: Recognizing and Treating Deficits." Noting the limited knowledge of many educators who find themselves to be the recipients of returning head-injured students, the authors provide a reprise of the cognitive-communicative deficits, classroom behaviors, and teaching strategies that may be most helpful to the HI students. Through text and a most helpful Appendix, readers will find the authors' considerable experience in this specialty area to be most effective.

As readers have earlier identified, "school" is the central core of a child's waking hours for many years. Thus, the structure of the classroom's demands, the teacher's requirements, and their peers' perception of the child with language disorders is of lasting influence. Language specialists can alleviate many of the difficulties and enhance a child's opportunities for success in this often alien setting. It is hoped that this text will help language professionals serve in a positive role. This role includes providing the most appropriate assessment possible.

REFERENCES

McCormick, E. (1993, September 6). Schoolkids increasingly troubled. *Monterey Herald.*

Westby, C., & Erickson, J. (1992). *Changing paradigms in language learning disabilities: The role of ethnography* (pp. v–viii). Gaithersburg, MD: Aspen Publishers.

—Katharine G. Butler, PhD
Editor, *Topics in Language Disorders*

Part I
Looking at Children in the School: Some Classroom Insights

Ethnography and classroom communication: Taking an "emic" perspective

Georgia Earnest García, PhD
Assistant Professor
Department of Curriculum and
*   Instruction*
Center for the Study of Reading
University of Illinois at
*   Urbana-Champaign*
Champaign, Illinois

Have you ever hurt
   about baskets?
I have, seeing my grandmother weaving
   for a long time.
Have you ever hurt about work?
I have, because my father works too hard
   and tells how he works.
Have you ever hurt about cattle?
I have, because my grandfather has been
   working on the cattle for a long time.
Have you ever hurt about school?
I have, because I learned a lot of words
   from my school,
And they are not my words (Anonymous; cited
in Cazden & Dickinson, 1981, p. 458)*

THIS POEM, written by an Apache child in Arizona, captures the focus of this article. A teacher in a kindergarten classroom in the Midwest also helped to

---

*Reprinted with permission from Cazden, C.B. & Dickinson, D.K. (1981). Language in education: Standardization versus cultural pluralism. In C.A. Ferguson & S.B. Heath (Eds). Language in the U.S.A. New York: Cambridge University Press. Copyright 1981, Cambridge University Press.

Top Lang Disord, 1992,12(3),54–66

set the tone for this article when she told me how she refers African American children to the school's speech-language pathologist (SLP), not because she suspects that the children are language delayed, but because she cannot understand them.

In this article, findings from ethnographic and microethnographic research are reviewed to further the understanding about how classroom interaction patterns can affect student achievement. This line of research should be of particular interest to SLPs and other special educators, not just because many of their referrals come from the classroom teacher, but because they are increasingly being called on to work within the classroom setting as part of the collaborative model of service delivery.

This article draws on findings from two research groups: (a) sociolinguists and classroom ethnographers who focus on understanding the role of language in classroom instruction and (b) educational anthropologists who study the cultural role of language in home, community, and school settings. After the concept of communicative competence, in general and in the classroom setting in particular, is discussed the findings from studies of home–school cultural discontinuities are reviewed to illustrate the importance of understanding the different norms that may govern language interactions in the home, community, and classroom. The article concludes by discussing how an *emic* perspective—the ability to empathize and understand other participants' perspectives and actions—can help teachers and clinicians bridge these differences between home and school.

COMMUNICATIVE COMPETENCE

Individuals are considered communicatively competent within a particular speech community when they know how to participate in socially appropriate ways (Florio-Ruane, 1987; Saville-Troike, 1989). *Communicative competence* is the knowledge that allows the individual to understand and act in concert with the expectations of the other participants. Young children learn how to communicate appropriately within the speech community in which they are raised. By the time they are five years old, most have acquired the linguistic and grammatical rudiments necessary to become competent speakers of the dialect and/or language heard around them (Lindfors, 1987). In addition to acquiring linquistic and grammatical rules, children become sensitive to the context, function, and meaning of interaction patterns. Depending on the speech community and one's role within that community, different ways of interacting and talking with parents, siblings, grandparents, other adults, and peers are learned (Saville-Troike, 1989).

Because communicative competence reflects what is appropriate in one speech community, there will be some variation in what is appropriate in a different speech community, even within the same country. These variations in communicative competence are called *sociolinguistic styles.* García, Pearson, and Jiménez (1990) point out that the "persistence of different sociolinguistic styles, even when children are exposed to the mass media and to universal schooling, suggests that these styles are acquired at an early age through socialization" (p. 54). It is likely that children's willingness to acquire new styles is affected by their motivation to participate not only in other speech communities but also in the larger society (see Ogbu & Matute-Bianchi, 1986).

Speech-language pathologists need to understand that children who speak a distinct dialect of English or who are learning English as a second language face problems that are different from those of a child who has not learned the appropriate sociolinguistic styles for his or her own speech community. In working with a dialect mismatch between the teacher and the child, the SLP needs to be sensitive to the fact that all English-speaking Americans speak a dialect of English, although some dialects are closer to standard English than others. Speech-language pathologists and classroom teachers need to understand that dialects, especially African American dialects, are not deviant forms of language (Labov, 1982). In fact, there is evidence that teachers' negative reactions to children's use of dialect, and not the children's use of dialect itself, is what appears to adversely affect their academic performance (García et al., 1990). Many children who speak a distinct dialect of English cease to participate when SLPs or teachers continually interrupt their speech to correct a dialect feature or insist that they only use standard English (García et al., 1990; Smitherman, 1986). Acquiring the type of standard English characteristic of written text is a relatively new task for all children. The task is eased, however, when the teacher shares the same dialect as the child or when the teacher is bidialectal and can help the child acquire two dialects (Delpit, 1988; Smitherman, 1986).

Children acquiring English as a second language are knowledgeable about appropriate ways of communicating in their native language but may need help in understanding and acquiring pragmatic skills in English. As an example, sixteen-year-old María, a Spanish-English bilingual student enrolled in a general equivalency degree (GED) program, appeared to be extremely fluent in both languages. Yet, she startled her adult education teacher when she authoritatively commanded that a worker at a McDonald's fast-food restaurant "give her" the food that she desired. Although the worker understood what

> *Children acquiring English as a second language are knowledgeable about appropriate ways of communicating in their native language but may need help in understanding and acquiring pragmatic skills in English.*

María had said, he was taken aback by her tone of voice and the imperative nature of her command. María had not acquired the appropriate courtesy protocol for this particular American social setting. Here is a situation in which the SLP and María's classroom teacher could work collaboratively to develop such activities as role playing or the use of videotapes to teach her the appropriate courtesy protocols in English.

Communicative competence encompasses knowledge about the linguistic features of language, the interaction patterns necessary to participate successfully in a variety of roles, and the cultural knowledge necessary to understand how communication (both verbal and nonverbal) is shaped and interpreted within a particular culture or speech community (Saville-Troike, 1989). Most adults have acquired communicative competence as young children immersed in the language and culture that surround them. Encountering new contexts of language use, children add to their communicative competence repertoire, increasing the sociolinguistic styles with which they are familiar.

CLASSROOM INTERACTION

The role that sociolinguistic styles play in determining school success may depend on the extent to which learning in the classroom is a function of the ability of the teacher and the child to sustain meaningful interaction in the classroom (see Gumperz, 1982; Leacock, 1972). A basic assumption underlying many of the current studies of classroom interaction is that teaching and learning are "interactive processes that require the active participation of teachers and students to ensure that information is conveyed as a precondition for learning" (Gumperz, 1982, p. 57).

Successful participation in the classroom requires a different type of communicative competence than that brought to school by most children (Cazden, 1988; Saville-Troike, 1989). The teacher's role and status differ from those of other adults with whom the child has interacted or continues to interact. For example, teachers tend to be more absolute in their authority, controlling not only how children verbally and nonverbally interact with them, but also how they interact with

other children. This is true both in traditional classrooms and in more open-ended whole language classrooms. Saville-Troike (1982) points out that communication in the American classroom traditionally has been characterized by "rigid turn-taking, with a raised hand to request a turn; [a definite] spacial arrangement, with children seated in rows of desks or around tables; and peer interaction which is initiated and controlled by adults" (p. 240). Although whole language classrooms provide students with more freedom (Goodman, 1989), the teacher still is the primary authority figure in the classroom. Children have to learn how to get the teacher's attention, when it is appropriate to speak to the teacher in private or in front of the group, how to respond appropriately, with whom they can interact and when, and what the different spacial arrangements are for the different activities.

Classroom discourse in traditional and whole language classrooms is characterized by identifiable patterns that students must learn if they are to acquire classroom communicative competence. For example, one of the most common patterns of classroom interaction in the United States occurs when the teacher initiates an interaction, the student responds, and the teacher evaluates the student's response (Cazden, 1988; Mehan, 1979). This pattern of interaction may occur in whole-class settings, in small group settings, or in teacher-student conferences. Teachers may use it to request an answer:

Teacher: John, what is the answer to #4?
John: Six.
Teacher: Good.

Other times, they may use it for clarification or to request unknown information:

Teacher: Diane, were you absent yesterday?
Diane: Uh-huh.
Teacher: Okay.

To avoid answering the question would be a breach of communicative conduct on the student's part. This pattern of interaction tends to characterize most teacher-led lessons, whether the lesson is reading, arithmetic, or social studies (Cazden, 1988). Teachers tend to use questions and answers within this pattern of interaction to elicit known information from children, so that they can monitor the children's comprehension of material and evaluate their performance (Cazden, 1988; Heath, 1982).

Throughout their interactions with children, teachers also use certain types of speech acts to control behavior and solicit cooperation. Because the functions of these acts may vary from one context to the other, children have to learn how to interpret their teacher's use of these acts (Sinclair & Coulthard, 1975). For example, it is not unusual for middle-class Anglo teachers (especially female teachers) to pose a command as a question (e.g., "John, will you please close the window?") (Delpit, 1988; Heath, 1982). Delpit (1988) points out that not all children are socialized in their speech communities to respond to this type of command. She contends that some African American children get into trouble in school because they respond to it literally, interpreting it as a request that can be denied and not a command.

Classroom activity also is characterized by routinized speech events, such as show and tell, taking roll, storybook time, round robin reading, and independent silent reading (Cazden, 1988; Saville-Troike, 1982).

Children learn to recognize these speech events by paying attention to the contextualization cues—verbal, paralinguistic, and kinesic behavior—that teachers routinely use to introduce them (Cazden, 1988; Gumperz, 1982). When children recognize the cues and are aware of the shifting activities or emphases that the cues represent, they are then free to focus on the content of the lesson (Cazden, 1988; Harker & Green, 1985).

Because many whole language teachers eschew telling students what to do, students in this type of classroom setting may need to rely more on their implicit understanding of classroom communicative competence and contextualization cues to understand the type of communicative behavior that is appropriate. For example, these students will need to know when the classroom activity has shifted and when it is appropriate to discuss information with a peer, call out information, wait for a turn, whisper, or be silent.

Children's entry into the classroom speech community is eased when children and their teachers participate in the same speech community outside the school (see Byers & Byers, 1972; Delpit, 1988; Heath, 1982; Michaels, 1981). In this situation, the teachers are familiar with the communicative competence that these children bring to school. As a result, they are able to shape these children's interactions, so that they become socialized into the school environment. When teachers are unfamiliar with the sociolinguistic styles of children, numerous opportunities for miscommunication and misassessment exist (Delpit, 1988; García, 1991; García et al., 1990; García & Pearson, 1991).

Classroom communicative competence

involves knowing and understanding the classroom rules that govern classroom interaction. Sometimes the rules are explicitly stated (e.g., "Raise your hand and wait to be called on before you talk."). Other times, they are implicit, and children must learn them through observation and trial and error, just as they acquire communicative competence in their speech community. Speech-language pathologists who collaborate with classroom teachers and work with children who are having difficulty interacting in the classroom need to understand the type of classroom communicative competence that the teacher expects. It also helps if the SLP is familiar with the type of communicative competence that the children are likely to bring with them to school. In this way, the SLP can help the teacher understand potential areas of miscommunication and help the child acquire the type of classroom communicative competence necessary to participate successfully in the classroom activities that the teacher deems necessary for instruction and evaluation.

HOME–SCHOOL DISCONTINUITIES

Differences in sociolinguistic styles in the American classroom have been noted in terms of participant structures (verbal and nonverbal patterns of interaction), discourse organizational patterns, and contextualization cues. Florio-Ruane (1987) points out that ethnographers who have contributed to this knowledge typically have studied home, school, and community settings through extensive participant observations and detailed analysis of recorded speech events. Their conclusions are the result of data triangulation—comparison and integration of data from a variety of sources—across home, community, and school settings.

Participant structures

Differences in the social conventions of verbal and nonverbal interaction can affect classroom teaching and learning. Who gets to speak when, how an individual holds the floor, and the way in which questions and answers are formulated and sequenced are aspects of communicative competence. As Hymes (1972) explains,

it is not that a child cannot answer questions but that questions and answers are defined in terms of one set of community norms rather than another, as to what counts as questions and answers, and as to what it means to be asked or to answer. (p. xxxi)

Findings from several ethnographic studies suggest that some children hold different expectations for their participation, which, if not accommodated by the teacher, may adversely affect their involvement in speech events that are an integral part of classroom instruction. For example, Philips (1972, 1983) found that Native American students from the Warm Springs Indian Reservation in Oregon did not willingly respond when the teachers solicited individual volunteers or when they called on students to respond as a group or

Who gets to speak when, how an individual holds the floor, and the way in which questions and answers are formulated and sequenced are aspects of communicative competence.

individually in front of the group. Students' participation level increased, however, when they interacted on a one-to-one basis with the teacher or when they participated in small groups directed by themselves. Interestingly, the latter participant structure paralleled the type of interaction that was most common for the students on the reservation.

Similar types of home–school discontinuities were reported by Boggs (1972, 1978) for Hawaiian dialect-speaking children, by Heath (1982) for African American children, and by Delgado-Gaitan (1987) for Mexican immigrant children. Boggs noted that the Hawaiian children in his study tended to respond as little as possible when a question was directed to them, but would not hesitate to blurt out the answer when the question was directed to another student or when the teacher directed the question to a group of students. This type of participant structure was similar to a discourse pattern, termed *talk story*, that was common in the children's speech community (see also Kawakami & Au, 1986).

Heath (1982) found that working-class African American students in the Carolina Piedmonts were not supposed to interact with their parents as conversational partners until they were considered "competent speakers." As a result, the children listened to adult conversation but did not actually participate in it. If an adult asked a child a question, it was one that required a "real" answer. Children learned to gain and hold the floor in their interactions with each other by using a story-starter style and analogies. Questions were not used to elicit known information for display purposes, the very type of question that most teachers use in the classroom to monitor and evaluate classroom learning.

Delgado-Gaitan (1987) discovered that Mexican immigrant children were more accustomed to a cooperative working environment than a competitive environment. At home, the children were allowed to negotiate how they would complete assigned tasks; whereas, at school, they were not. When the children tried to work cooperatively at school, the teacher misinterpreted their actions, viewing their efforts as cheating or disruptive.

Because classroom communication involves "the language of curriculum, the language of control, and the language of personal identity" (Cazden, 1988, p. 3), cultural discontinuities between home and school can result in lost teaching and learning opportunities, as well as incorrect assessment of children's capabilities (see García & Pearson, 1991). Speech-language pathologists, psychologists, special educators, and classroom teachers need to be aware of the social context of the testing situation, regardless of whether it is a formal or informal setting. Leap (1982), for example, found that a Native American student hardly responded when she was asked to retell a story read in class. She produced an extensive narrative, however, when she was asked to make up a story about a classmate's picture. Edwards and García (1989) also discovered that an African American child, who was labeled language delayed by the classroom teacher, was very verbal but reticent to participate in adult–child storybook interactions because these interactions did not characterize her home life.

Discourse organization patterns

Cultural differences in how students structure their speech and writing also have been documented. Several study findings suggest that teachers do not always understand why some groups of students may structure their oral speech in ways that vary from the classroom norm (Cooley & Lujan, 1982; Michaels, 1981). For example, Cooley and Lujan explored why college instructors said that their Native American students, who also happened to be monolingual English speakers, tended to ramble when they gave formal presentations in class. Through a comparative analysis, these researchers found that the structure and the content of the Native American students' oral speeches tended to parallel those of their tribal elders. Both groups structured their speeches so that several topics were introduced in sequence without much transition, although coreferencing helped to provide cohesion within the topics. The students also tended to emphasize their sources of information more than the information itself, a characteristic of Native American culture.

Michaels (1981) found differences in discourse patterns among Anglo and African American first graders during sharing time. The Anglo children tended to use a topic-centered style, whereas the African American children used a topic-associating style that consisted of a series of "implicitly associated personal anecdotes" (p. 429). There were no explicit statements of overall themes or points, but the anecdotes all related to a particular topic or theme that had to be inferred. Topic shifts were signaled prosodically and appeared to be difficult for the teacher to follow. The end result was that the Anglo teacher was able to use questions to shape the Anglo children's narratives, helping them to approximate the type of decontextualized, orderly sequenced prose that she thought they would later encounter in their reading. The teacher's attempts to help the African American children, however, were mistimed and inappropriate. She eventually stopped calling on these children because she could not understand the focus of their presentations.

Contextualization cues

The importance of contextualization cues in forming the content and surface style of interaction in the classroom should not be overlooked. Contextualization cues can include formulaic expressions; code, dialect, and style switching; prosodic signs, such as gaze direction, proxemic distance, and kinesic rhythm or timing; choices among lexical and syntactic options; phonetic and rhythmic signs; and conversational openings, closings, and sequencings (Erickson & Shultz, 1977; Gumperz, 1982). As Gumperz explains, these cues allow the activity to be interpreted, "the semantic content to be understood, and the relationship of each sentence to the next to be foreseen" (p. 31). When a listener does not perceive a cue or does not know its function, misunderstandings and different interpretations may occur. In the classroom this may result in misinterpretation of behavior and loss of feedback.

Gumperz (1982) suggests that misinterpretation of contextualization cues in the classroom especially may occur because children use stress, rhythm, and intonation to communicate what adults customarily might put into words. For example, African American children he studied in Berkeley tended to respond to the teachers' requests for action or information by saying, "I don't know," "I can't read," "I don't want to do this," or "I can't do this." The teachers' usual response was to ignore the children or to halt any further interaction. An analysis of the contextualized cues used by the students, however, revealed "similar intonational structures, characterized by a high pitch register, sustained tone, and vowel elongation on the last syllable" (p. 19). When a panel of African American adults reviewed the speech samples, they said that the children actually were saying that they did not like to work alone and needed help.

Differences in the timing of nonverbal gestures also have been noted. For example, Byers and Byers (1972) discovered that an Anglo teacher did not maintain the same type of eye contact with her Anglo children as she did with her African American children. Although the African American children and Anglo teacher actually gazed at each other more often than did the teacher and Anglo children, their pauses were mistimed. As a result, less eye contact was realized. Byers and Byers suggest that differences in contextualization cues may mean that students will miss "subtle interconnections" in the presentation of information. As a result, students will not feel secure "in what [they have] learned and in what the significance of learning is" (p. 27).

There are several reasons why children and teachers from different speech communities may miscommunicate. Home–school discontinuities may be reflected in different participant structures, discourse organization patterns, and contextualization cues. Clinicians need to be aware of these differences and take the time to find out whether a child's communication problem represents such a discontinuity. To do this, they will need to observe both the teacher and the child in the classroom, documenting the points of miscommunication and the type of classroom communicative competence that the teacher expects. In addition, they will have to find out more about the child's background and the type of communicative competence that prevails in the child's speech community. They especially need to be open to input from the child's parents and other members of the community. Heath (1982) began her longitudinal study of literacy and communicative behavior in the Carolina Piedmonts when the African American children's parents told her that they did not understand why the teachers said that their children could not answer questions. Juxtaposing conflicting points of information is one way to discover home–school discontinuities that have the potential for successful resolutions.

BRIDGING DIFFERENCES

Several researchers and educators have suggested that school professionals (classroom teachers, SLPs, special educators, administrators, and psychologists) need to be aware of the emic perspective. That is, they need to understand the importance of viewing school events from the cultural perspectives of the participants. To do this, these professionals not only have to be open to understanding how communicative events are interpreted by others, but also have to acknowledge that their own patterns of interaction are influenced by their own socialization. A key component of the emic perspective is the ability to observe others from their perspective and to understand how one is conditioned by one's own perspective.

Educators who have been willing to bridge differences in communicative competence have met with some success. For example, the Kamehameha Early Education Program (KEEP) in Hawaii (Au, 1980) has had considerable success in increasing Hawaiian children's reading comprehension by allowing the students to engage in the type of talk story that Boggs (1972,

---

A key component of the emic perspective is the ability to observe others from their perspective and to understand how one is conditioned by one's own perspective.

1978) described. Although teachers in the KEEP program generally initiate reading comprehension questions, the students respond by calling out their answers and building on each other's responses until the group as a whole has reacted to the teachers' questions. The interaction pattern that dominates during this part of the instruction is quite different from the teacher initiates–student responds–teacher evaluates type of pattern that generally characterizes most reading group instruction.

Two other examples are provided by Heath (1982) and Erickson and Mohatt (1982). In Heath's study (1982), the teach-

ers were able to bridge differences in interaction patterns by incorporating more of the African American students' questioning patterns in their own classroom instruction and by attempting to introduce the African American students, in a risk-free manner, to the types of questions that they preferred. Erickson and Mohatt (1982) found that an Anglo teacher was able to interact successfully with his Native American students when he accommodated to cultural differences in sociolinguistic styles throughout the year by increasing his one-on-one interactions with the students and reducing the "spotlighting" of student interactions in front of an audience.

Many times observant teachers will naturally adjust to what they perceive to be a lack of communication. Other times, they will need to rely on outside help to explain a classroom occurrence they do not understand. Carrasco (1981) found that even a well-intentioned bilingual teacher misread the potential capability of one of her bilingual students. In response to a bilingual aide's comment that the Latino children talked more often in groups, Carrasco began to videotape one of the bilingual children whom the teacher was considering retaining. He found that this child was the one who was helping the other students complete work that the teacher did not think she could do on her own.

Genishi (1985) points out that teachers frequently may not be able to do systematic observations because of the nature of their jobs. Clinicians should be able to help teachers in this area. The clinician may be able to discover why communication has gone awry by observing or videotaping (or both) the classroom; interviewing the teacher, the child, and the child's parents; and visiting the child's home and community. The clinician can share this information with the classroom teacher and use what she or he knows about language acquisition, classroom communicative competence, and potential home–school discontinuities (see Harker & Green, 1985) to help the teacher develop a plan to bridge communication differences.

Sometimes, bridging communication differences may involve a radical change in how the teacher presents material or facilitates interaction, such as found in the KEEP program (Au, 1980). Other times, it may involve a simple change, such as not interrupting the oral reading of a dialect-speaking student when the student uses a dialect feature that preserves meaning, or becoming aware of how students from a particular speech community use language, as described by Gumperz (1982). Still other times, it may involve an instructional modification, in which the teacher modifies the ways in which she or he elicits students' active participation in a communicative event deemed necessary for learning and instruction, at the same time that he or she makes explicit, or introduces students to, those aspects of classroom communicative competence that tend to prevail in the American classroom, as in Heath (1982).

•   •   •

If school professionals are to take an emic perspective, in which the focus is on understanding the situation from the different cultural perspectives of the participants, they need to step out of their roles as participants in the school's speech community. They need to recognize that there are other patterns of communication that are just as viable as those they are accustomed to in school. School professionals also have to be willing to search for alternative explanations when children are not performing well in school. They have to be willing to accept the interpretations and the observations of not just the teacher, but also of the child, the child's parents, and the community members.

The clinician can help in this effort. By using ethnographic techniques, such as home–school observation, interviews, and data triangulation, the clinician can determine whether a communication problem is due to a mismatch between the child's communicative competence and the classroom communicative competence expected at school. An ethnographic approach not only can help clinicians understand the source of communication problems, but also can help them work with the classroom teacher, the student, and the student's parents to design a plan, so that differences in communicative competence can be bridged.

REFERENCES

Au, K.H.-P. (1980). Participation structures in a reading lesson with Hawaiian children: Analysis of culturally appropriate instructional events. *Anthropology and Education Quarterly, 11,* 91–115.

Boggs, S.T. (1972). The meaning of questions and narratives to Hawaiian children. In C.B. Cazden, V.P. John, & D. Hymes (Eds.), *Functions of language in the classroom* (pp. 299–327). New York: Teachers College Press.

Boggs, S.T. (1978). The development of verbal disputing in part-Hawaiian children. *Language in Society, 7,* 325–344.

Byers, P. & Byers, B. (1972). In C.B. Cazden, V.P. John, & D. Hymes (Eds.), *Functions of language in the classroom* (pp. 3–31). New York: Teachers College Press.

Carrasco, R.L. (1981). Expanded awareness of student performance: A case study in applied ethnographic monitoring in a bilingual classroom. In H.T. Trueba, G.P. Guthrie, & K.H. Au (Eds.), *Culture and the bilingual classroom: Studies in classroom ethnography* (pp. 153–177). Rowley, MA: Newbury House.

Cazden, C.B. (1988). *Classroom discourse: The language of teaching and learning.* Portsmouth, NH: Heinemann.

Cazden, C.B. & Dickinson, D.K. (1981). Language in education: Standardization versus cultural pluralism. In C.A. Ferguson & S.B. Heath (Eds.), *Language in the USA* (pp. 446–468). New York: Cambridge University Press.

Cooley, D., & Lujan, P. (1982). A structural analysis of speeches by Native American students. In F. Barkin, E.A. Brandt, & J. Ornstein-Galicia (Eds.), *Bilingualism and language contact: Spanish, English, and Native American languages* (pp. 80–92). New York: Teachers College Press.

Delgado-Gaitan, C. (1987). Traditions and transitions in the learning process of Mexican children: An ethnographic view. In G. Spindler & L. Spindler (Eds.) *Interpretive ethnography of education: At home and abroad* (pp. 333–359). Hillsdale, NJ: Erlbaum.

Delpit, L. (1988). The silenced dialogue: Power and pedagogy in educating other people's children. *Harvard Educational Review, 58*(3), 280–298.

Edwards, P.A., & García, G.E. (1989, November). *A case study of one low-income mother learning to share books with her four-year-old daughter.* Paper presented at the National Reading Conference, Austin, TX.

Erickson, F., & Mohatt, G. (1982). Cultural organization of participation structures in two classrooms of Indian students. In G. Spindler (Ed.), *Doing the ethnography of schooling: Educational anthropology in action* (pp. 132–174). Orlando, FL: Holt, Rinehart & Winston.

Erickson, F., & Shultz, J. (1977). When is a context? Some issues and methods in the analysis of social competence. *The Quarterly Newsletter of the Institute for Comparative Human Development, 1,* 5–9.

Florio-Ruane, S. (1987). Sociolinguistics for educational researchers. *American Educational Research Journal, 24*(2), 185–197.

García, G.E. (1991). Factors influencing the English reading test performance of Spanish-speaking Hispanic children. *Reading Research Quarterly, 23*(4), 371–392.

García, G.E., & Pearson, P.D. (1991). The role of assessment in a diverse society. In E. Hiebert (Ed.), *Literacy in a diverse society: Perspectives, practices, and policies* (pp. 253–278). New York: Teachers College Press.

García, G.E., Pearson, P.D., & Jiménez, R.T. (1990). *The at-risk dilemma: A synthesis of reading research* (study 2.2.3.3b). Urbana-Champaign, IL: University of Illinois, Reading Research & Education Center.

Genishi, C. (1985). Observing communicative performance in young children. In A. Jagger & M.T. Smith-Burke (Eds.), *Observing the language learner* (pp. 131–142). Newark, DE: International Reading Association; and Urbana, IL: National Council of Teachers of English.

Goodman, K.S. (1989). Whole language research: Foundations and development. *The Elementary School Journal, 90*(2), 207–221.

Gumperz, J. (1982). *Discourse strategies: Studies in interactional sociolinguistics I.* New York: Cambridge University Press.

Harker, J.O., & Green, J.L. (1985). When you get the right answer to the wrong question: Observing and understanding communication in classrooms. In A. Jagger & M.T. Smith-Burke (Eds.), *Observing the language learner* (pp. 221–231). Newark, DE: International Reading Association; and Urbana, IL: National Council of Teachers of English.

Heath, S.B. (1982). Questioning at school and at home: A comparative study. In G. Spindler (Ed.), *Doing the ethnography of schooling: Educational anthropology in action* (pp. 102–131). Orlando, FL: Holt, Rinehart & Winston.

Hymes, D. (1972). Introduction. In C.B. Cazden, V.P. John, & D. Hymes (Eds.), *Functions of language in the classroom.* New York: Teachers College Press.

Kawakami, A.J., & Au, K.H.-P. (1986). Encouraging reading and language development in cultural minority children. *Topics in Language Disorders, 6*(2), 71–80.

Labov, W. (1982). Objectivity and commitment in linguistic science. The case of the Black English trial in Ann Arbor. *Language in Society, 11,* 165–201.

Leacock, E.B. (1972). Abstract versus concrete speech: A false dichotomy. In C.B. Cazden, V.P. John, & D. Hymes (Eds.), *Functions of language in the classroom* (pp. 111–134). New York: Teachers College Press.

Leap, W.L. (1982). The study of Indian English in the U.S. Southwest: Retrospect and prospect. In F. Barkin, E.A. Brandt, & J. Ornstein-Galicia (Eds.), *Bilingualism and language contact: Spanish, English and Native American languages* (pp. 101–119). New York: Teachers College Press.

Lindfors, J.W. (1987). *Children's language and learning* (2nd ed.). Englewood Cliffs, NJ: Prentice-Hall.

Mehan, H. (1979). *Learning lessons.* Cambridge: Harvard University Press.

Michaels, S. (1981). Sharing time: Children's narrative styles and differential access to literacy. *Language in Society, 10,* 423–442.

Ogbu, J.U., & Matute-Bianchi, M.E. (1986). Understanding sociocultural factors: Knowledge, identity, and school adjustment. In *Beyond language: Social and cultural factors in schooling language minority students* (pp.

73–142). (Compiled by California State Department of Education.) Los Angeles: Evaluation, Dissemination & Assessment Center.

Philips, S. (1972). Participant structures and communicative competence: Warm Springs children in community and classroom. In C.B. Cazden, V.P. John, & D. Hymes (Eds.), *Functions of language in the classroom* (pp. 370–394. New York: Teachers College Press.

Philips, S. (1983). *The invisible culture: Communication in classroom and community on the Warm Springs Indian Reservation.* White Plains, NY: Longman.

Saville-Troike, M. (1982). *The ethnography of communication: An introduction* (1st ed.). Baltimore: University Park Press.

Saville-Troike, M. (1989). *The ethnography of communication: An introduction* (2nd ed.). New York: Basil Blackwell.

Sinclair, J. McH., & Coulthard, R.M. (1975). *Toward an analysis of discourse: The English used by teachers and pupils.* London: Oxford University Press.

Smitherman, G. (1986). *Talkin and testifyin: The language of Black America.* Detroit: Wayne State University.

Whole language in context: Insights into the current great debate

Diane J. Sawyer, PhD
Murfree Professor of Dyslexic Studies
Elementary and Special Education
Middle Tennessee State University
Murfreesboro, Tennessee

I used to think reading was making sense of a story but now I know it is just letters.
Amy Anderson, age 6 (Michel, 1990, p. 43)

With this simple reflection on her learning, Amy lays bare one of the significant issues that distinguishes the whole language approach to beginning reading experiences from the traditional approaches popular in the United States throughout much of our history. The focus of instruction for beginning reading has been the letters, sounds, words, and punctuation that comprise the pages of text. Meaning was viewed as attainable only when all of these fragments were skillfully reassembled by the reader. Learning to recognize and to associate these fragments, one with another and all in concert, can become a laborious and confusing process. In addition, as may be inferred from Amy's comment, some children lose sight of the goal along the way. Some falter and others fail altogether to acquire reading proficiency.

Top Lang Disord, 1991,11(3),1–13
© 1991 Aspen Publishers, Inc.

These children become tangled in the intricacies of content (what they must learn about the way print codes meaning) and the complexity of instructional vehicles—the workbooks and drill sheets and management techniques teachers have used to carve up and deliver the content. This is what some of Amy's classmates came to understand about reading after a few months of immersion in traditional first-grade reading instruction: "Reading is stand up, sit down." "Reading is marking x's and circles." (Michel, 1990, p. 43).

On the other side of the world, New Zealand children over the past decade have been learning to read in a different way. Language-based beginning reading experiences in New Zealand maintain the focus on meaning at all times. Children are encouraged to use their own background knowledge and information from the title, pictures, and earlier portions of a story to anticipate or predict what might reasonably be coded on a page. More global cueing systems—pictures, syntax, and semantics—give way to graphophonic or letter–sound cues only when a reasonable estimate of the printed message cannot be developed in any other way (Mooney, 1988). Thus, constructing meaning from minimal cues is the prime focus of New Zealand instruction. Accuracy in naming printed words is viewed as only one means for obtaining meaning. Miscalled words are understood as *miscues*, the consequence of misinterpreting cues attended to in the process of making sense of the story. If the miscalling does not affect meaning (e.g., saying *a* for *the*), teacher and reader tend to ignore it and proceed. When meaning is affected, rereading (to examine previously noted and possibly

additional cues) is encouraged as a means of recovering meaning and effectively continuing with the process of predicting and constructing further meaning. Unlike Amy, preschoolers' expectations that reading involves making sense of a story are not denied in the course of instruction. New Zealand enjoys a 99% literacy rate.

The language-based, meaning-driven instructional approach used in New Zealand has come to be known in the United States as the whole language approach, giving rise to questions about the whole language movement: How does whole language instruction, overall, differ from traditional reading practices in the United States? What are the implications of the whole language movement for identifying and serving language/reading-impaired students? These questions guided development of this article.

HISTORY OF U.S. READING INSTRUCTION

Since the colonial period of American history, beginning reading instruction has focused on teaching the alphabet, syllables, and words. From the hornbook, imported from England in the 1600s, to the primers, including the New England Primer (1683), and a host of readers, including Webster's Blue Back Speller during the 1700s and early 1800s, beginning reading stressed memorization of letter names and the spelling of common syllables and words.

In the mid-1800s, reading instruction in the United States began to be questioned in light of the work of Pestalozzi. (Smith, 1986) In principle, Pestalozzi advocated what, today, might be called a multisensory approach. Children attended to pictures of word referents (e.g., house), watched as the word was written, traced the form in the air, copied the word, sounded out the letters and blended the sounds into the whole spoken word (Smith, 1986). Content was ordered, simple to complex, and much opportunity for practice was provided. Child involvement and word meaning was in focus for the first time. Comprehension questions began to appear in materials for older readers.

Emphasis on meaning soon led to the development of new series of reading books wherein words, as whole units, provided the entrée to reading in the latter half of the 19th century (Smith, 1986). Following this introduction through meaning, instruction then moved to learning the alphabet and sounds as before. The alphabetic-phonics materials, with their emphasis on letters, syllables, and sounds to introduce reading, remained popular throughout the latter half of the century. The most familiar example of these was the McGuffey Readers.

At the turn of the century, attention turned to the content of children's reading materials. Primers and readers had previously relied heavily on religious, moral, patriotic, or scientific content. In the 1890s, Herbart, a German philosopher, urged the inclusion of good literature in the curriculum. Eliot, president of Harvard University, suggested the use of literature in

---

At the turn of the century, attention turned to the content of children's reading materials.

---

place of specially prepared reading books. In fact, his comments (cited in Smith, 1986) could easily be attributed to whole language enthusiasts today:

It would be for the advancement of the whole public school system if every reader were hereafter to be absolutely excluded from the school. I object to them because they are not real literature; they are but scraps of literature, even when the single lessons or materials of which they are composed are taken from literature. (p. 120)

Then, as today, there was considerable interest in developing appreciation for, and life-long interest in, literature. Then, as today, reading for meaning occupied center stage in the academic theater. At about this time also, silent independent reading of trade books, oral sharing of favorite segments, and distributing of multiple copies of some trade books for use during this sharing time were recommended. Such activities characterize reading in whole language classrooms today, especially at third grade and beyond.

Between 1910 and 1930, reading was increasingly viewed as a process to derive meaning, and silent reading as the preferred mode of practice came to the fore. As a means of checking on silent reading, publishers began to produce seatwork materials eliciting responses, of various types, related to text read silently. Such materials proliferated in the decades that followed.

Even though attention during the first 3 decades of this century seemed to focus on meaning, mastery of the mechanics of reading (phonics or whole word recognition) was still viewed as the primary focus for beginning reading. While the eventual goal of reading was acknowledged to be apprehension of the message and appreciation of the form of the message, attaining those goals was seen to be dependent on first mastering the code.

During the decades spanning 1930 to 1960, the use of phonics for initial instruction in the code declined. Whole words, phrases, and sentences along with chart stories based on children's own experiences dominated early first-grade instruction. Phonic elements were taught later in first grade and beyond. Use of structural analysis and context clues as additional strategies for word recognition were introduced (Smith, 1986). Also during this period, reading began to be viewed within the context of all the language arts. The importance of effective communication through listening, speaking, reading, and writing began to be emphasized. The most fundamental premise of the current whole language movement is that of concomitant development in all of the language arts.

By 1960, practices involving beginning reading instruction were almost equally divided between phonics and the whole word approach. The Columbia-Carnegie Study of Reading Research and Its Communication (cited in Smith, 1986) reported that "Some sort of phonics is universal—and so is some sort of whole-word method." (p. 351) That is, 90% of the first-grade classes surveyed were taught new words as whole units on half or more of the days, and 82% of the classes were taught to sound out words from letters and letter combinations on half or more of the days.

However, in 1968, Jeanne Chall published her report, *Learning to Read: The Great Debate*. She had reviewed available research studies in an attempt to document the relative effectiveness of phonics versus the whole word approach. Her review suggested a slight edge for phonics. For many publishers, this report and its wide acceptance among professional reading educators offered sufficient support to reemphasize early and sustained phonics instruction in subsequent editions of basal readers. It was not until the mid-1980s that widespread dissatisfaction with reading instruction was again apparent. Concern was precipitated by continuing reports of generally unacceptable levels of reading performance among U.S. school children (National Assessment of Educational Progress, 1985).

At about the same time, a growing body of research was documenting that reading involves active participation of the reader in a complex of perceptual and cognitive processes. Intensive research on the reading process during the 1970s led to the construction of models to explain decoding (e.g., LaBerge & Samuels, 1974) and comprehension (e.g., Kintsch & Van Dijk, 1978; Rumelhart, 1977) as well as the characteristics of readers, text, and task that affect the products of both (Mosenthal, 1984). (See Westby & Costlow, "Implementing a Whole Language Program in a Special Education Class," this issue.) Reader experiences, text structure, and situational conditions, including the task to be accomplished, were now understood to interact. Instructional approaches were predicated on the assumption that to learn to read and write, one needed to learn content; letters, sounds, words, and print conventions could no longer be defended. The time was ripe for a paradigm shift from product, or what to learn, to process, or how to learn.

INSTRUCTIONAL APPROACHES AND LEARNING PROCESSES

The traditional basal reader approach to beginning reading instruction, whether beginning with whole words, phonics, or a combination, embodies the traditional view that code mastery is a precondition for reading for meaning. This part-to-whole view of reading probably originated in armchair introspection. Adult readers considered what they did when they read and set about to teach others what they reasoned to be the appropriate sequence of actions. In fact, the first scientific research methodology applied in the field of psychology involved such introspection. Advocated by Wundt (cited in Snelbecker, 1974) in the late 1800s, this was called the "science of experience."

It is behavioral psychology, however, with its emphasis on analysis of behavior as a response to some precipitating stimulus, that is likely responsible for the content and practices advocated in basal reading series over the last century. Founded by Watson at the turn of the century, this school of thought theorized that, through learning, an organism developed increasingly effective means for coping with the environment (Snelbecker, 1974).

Behaviorism is rooted in the belief that behavior is controlled by its consequences. Learning comes about as one seeks pleasure and avoids pain. Behaviorists viewed learners as relatively passive and subject to the forces at work in the environment. People do not control the world but are controlled by it.

The behaviorist view was extended and elaborated on by the connectionist theories of Thorndike (cited in Snelbecker, 1974, p. 65), who viewed the product of learning as situation-response connections. That is, learning disposed one habitually to respond in a particular way given a specific situation.

Building on the work of Thorndike and Pavlov, Skinner substantially refined behaviorist learning theory (Perkinson, 1984). Skinner studied changes in behavior as a consequence of experimental manipulation of conditions. From Skinner's point of view, there were no inner causes of human behavior; there were no needs, drives, motives, or anything else "inside the skin" (Perkinson, 1984, p. 74) that explained human behavior. He maintained that events and conditions in the world shaped behavior.

Applied to learning to read, the theories of Thorndike and Skinner led to analyzing the act into minute elements of decoding and comprehension. Each piece was then presented in isolation, and repeated appropriate responses were rewarded with praise, stars, and, rather recently, happy-face stickers. It was expected that these isolated behaviors would be strung together by the child into performance of a fully integrated act. Sight–word recognition, phonics knowledge, blending, subject recognition, awareness of sequence, and other skills would, eventually, coalesce into functional reading behavior. This approach to reading instruction has come to be known as the *bottom-up* or *outside-in* view because the external and artificial tasks must be internalized by the individual and become a well-orchestrated personal response to a specific condition or stimulating event in the environment. Criticism leveled against this theory of learning is that the fragments are presented in isolation, in arbitrary sequence, outside the bounds of either meaning or specific goals that could facilitate organization, orchestration, and integration of a thoughtful response to print.

In contrast, the whole language movement might trace its roots to Dewey's functionalism. Functionalism considered learning to be a process wherein the mind mediates between the environment and the needs of the organism (Snelbecker, 1974). Within this view of learning, the learner takes a more active part. Dewey viewed learning as the process of acquiring behaviors that permitted one to function successfully in the environment. For Dewey, experiences in the world turned native intelligence into the power to control the environment. (Monroe, 1950)

Perhaps the strongest influence on the whole language movement, by far, originates in the field of cognitive psychology. Cognitivists view learning as a process, not a product. Emphasis is on the active learner who personally selects and organizes experiences in a situation and constructs understandings of situations and events. The emphasis is on learning as the learner experiences it rather than on conditions in the environment that might precipitate learning (Snelbecker, 1974). Learning thus involves the application of complex intellectual abilities to interpret a situation in light of what has been previously learned, and to modify previous knowledge to the extent that is necessary, in light of the new situation. Knowledge is not simply transmitted by a teacher and taken in, in total, by the learner.

According to cognitive construct theorists, ". . . the major task of the instructor is to provide whatever guidance seems nec-essary [for children] in a meaningful way." (Snelbecker, 1974, p. 432) In addition, "to organize new information instructional materials or the directions provided by the teacher should [contain] some means whereby the student can develop skills in evaluating his own progress." (Snelbecker, 1974, p. 432).

Two other early theorists, whose developmental/constructivist views have undoubtedly influenced the whole language movement, are Bartlett and Piaget. Bartlett's (1932) early work on memory led him to propose that knowledge is stored in organized systems of information called schemata. A schema for dog, for example, probably is not built up by carefully presenting only one piece of the dog at a time until the whole is fully assembled. Rather, dog comes to be understood through many experiences with the whole dog in different contexts.

Piaget's work in child development added to Bartlett's theory regarding schemata. Piaget asserted that children learn through their experiences but that they personally organize their experiences into an understanding of the world (cited in Furth, 1969). Children make meaning. Even more importantly, Piaget asserted that cognitive development, the consequence of learning, occurs in hierarchical stages. Successive stages of competencies depend on and grow out of the concepts and understandings about the world that were developed during the previous stages. What children learn and how they learn in new situations at least partly depends on the framework of knowledge and experiences that is already in place to support new learning. Provided with rich experiences, children naturally abstract the pertinent details they are ready to attend to and work out an understanding of, and build into schemata or systems of understandings about the world.

It is these views of the learning process, in combination, that undergirds the whole language movement. The whole language approach is a *top-down* or *inside-out* view wherein learning is driven by the learner and involves the highly personal and individual linking of what is known to what is new. This explains incomplete learning, misinterpretations, and errors, as well as creative and insightful interpretations of information and experiences. Whole language tenets and practices offer a rationale and means for implementing process-based instruction.

WHOLE LANGUAGE VIEW OF LITERACY ACQUISITION

Although an emphasis on meaning and use of whole literature selections receives wide attention, this is not, as the historical overview pointed out, newly advocated by the whole language movement. Further, these are not the most critical distinctions between whole language and other approaches. The whole language approach builds on three basic tenets of language learning:

1. Children acquire language through immersion in a language-rich envi-

---

Whole language tenets and practices offer a rationale and means for implementing process-based instruction.

---

ronment (e.g., Chomsky, 1957; Clark, 1973; Weaver, 1988).

2. Language learning is directed by the child to accomplish personal communication goals (Halliday, 1975).

3. Parents and other supportive adults assist in this learning process by providing models through personal communication with others, and by listening carefully and responding appropriately to communication attempts by children.

Offering questions and restatements to assist in expression and to verify intended content of the messages aids children in acquiring increasingly more effective communication and increasingly more adult forms of expression (Wells, 1986).

Learning language in the home, family, and community contexts is now understood to be a transactional process. A transaction involves cooperation among individuals in order to reach a goal. In learning language, children are not specifically taught what to say, when to say it, or how to say it. Instead, parents and other adults question children when something is not clear and then paraphrase to check the accuracy of their interpretations of the intended messages. As observers and participants, young children learn to use words (vocabulary) and word order (syntax) as well as intonation, gestures, and facial expression to convey meaning. When a message they want to convey cannot be understood, a parent usually helps the child negotiate the complexities of word choice, word order, and idea sequencing in order to make the message clear. Parents ask questions, supply a possible sentence, and make bridging statements. Parents become the child's partners in communication, and from this supportive modeling the child learns how to become a more effective communicator.

The driving force behind the whole language approach is the belief that children can acquire literacy in much the same way they acquired spoken language. Given experiences in observing the role of the reader and writer, and given assistance in negotiating the tasks involved in taking on the role personally, children will acquire literacy as effectively and efficiently as they acquire language. The whole language approach is an attempt to apply the transactional process observed in language learning to the process of literacy acquisition. Reading and writing are also language acts. It is reasonable to suppose that children can acquire competence in these areas given immersion in a literate environment, opportunities to communicate through print, and supportive feedback in a transactional context. This is the foundation of the whole language philosophy.

In whole language classrooms, children engage in activities that help them to use language, in all its forms, to express meaning, and to understand others and the world. Children learn to read and write by participating in reading and writing activities, using whatever skills and resources they possess at that time, to communicate through print. Activities that are personally meaningful to the child are essential, for in grappling with a personal need to express and to understand, children will acquire the necessary knowledge, rules, and conventions to accomplish their goals. In whole language classrooms, the teacher takes on the role of the supportive adult who attends closely to the child's commu-

nication intentions and provides specific support, in a partnering relationship, to accomplish the goal.

The challenge for whole language teachers is great, for contrary to the popular view, instruction in the content and strategies for effective reading and writing must be provided. However, different children require somewhat different information and strategies at different times. Teachers must learn to become effective observers of individual children and sophisticated interpreters of their communication efforts. Teachers must provide direct instruction in specific reading and writing skills, including sound and symbol correspondences and whole words, when a child demonstrates readiness to respond and internalize it. This challenge for the whole language teacher is especially critical when working with language/learning disabled students whose competencies develop unevenly.

Direct instruction in whole language classrooms should be consistent with what Vygotsky (1962) describes as the child's "zone of proximal development." This refers to the organization of knowledge, skills, and interests, at any given time, that establishes the most receptive climate for specific new learning from teacher or peers. What should be taught, to whom, and when, depends on the teachers' and language specialists' perceptions of the skills needed to grasp or convey effectively a given message, and children's current status with regard to those skills.

Few teachers have had adequate experiences in assessing texts, readers, and tasks as noted above. Teachers have, instead, been trained to deliver prepackaged lessons from basal reading manuals. As a consequence, in many classrooms where whole language practices are said to be underway, we might see modeling of reading and writing behaviors by teachers, and many opportunities for student engagement in reading and writing. However, specific guidance to help each child personally apply knowledge possessed and strategies observed is often lacking. In fact, far too many new converts to whole language presume that the motivation to read and write, in and of itself, will carry a child through the process of skill acquisition virtually independent of the teacher. Unfortunately, observing someone else apply a strategy or discuss a bit of knowledge about the reading process is not sufficient to adopt the strategy or knowledge for personal use in a new situation. Direct teaching is critical in helping children to achieve new levels of independence in reading and writing. We have every reason to expect that limited progress and failure will be evident when whole language techniques are not accompanied by direct instruction. In effective whole language classrooms, direct teaching is provided always in the context of valid activities that involve getting or expressing meaning.

PROMOTING LITERATE BEHAVIOR

In whole language classrooms, trade books and materials for writing and drawing are the materials used for instruction. In all situations, getting or conveying meaning is always the primary focus. Four different types of activities are used to keep focus on meaning while providing opportunities to model the reader's and writer's tasks, to teach specific content and strategies, and to practice assuming the reader's and writer's role. These vehicles are (a) reading to or writing with children, (b) shared reading, (c) guiding children's reading or conferencing about their writing, and (d) independent reading or writing. (See Mooney, 1988; Department of Education, 1985; Atwell, 1987 for more detail.)

Reading aloud to children or writing experience stories with them offers teachers the opportunity to model consciously the task of the reader or writer in a valid context. This parallels the oral language modeling of adults during the language acquisition period. Through reading to or writing with children, they acquire a sense of how books work, the style of book language, a feel for colorful language and new vocabulary, and an awareness of different ways of organizing to say something. There is a great emphasis on this vehicle during kindergarten and early first grade, but it tapers off after second grade.

Shared reading, a technique developed by Holdaway (1979), is the opportunity for children to join in with the teacher in reading a familiar passage or story. Through this activity, the teacher explicitly demonstrates what a reader must do to grasp an author's message. Using enlarged texts, or multiple copies, such basics as directionality, how to respond to different punctuation, how to use pictures and text together, and how to work through the pronunciation or meaning of an unfamiliar word or the meaning of an uncommon sentence structure are demonstrated. (See Weaver, "Whole Language and Its Potential for Developing Readers," this issue.) Shared reading is more frequently engaged during kindergarten and first grade, but some shared book experiences may be found at all elementary grade levels. We might liken this activity to adults who adjust their language form and complexity when directly addressing a young child to ensure that their language is consistent with the child's level of competence to understand and respond.

In guided reading and in conferencing about writing in progress, children take the reins and assume responsibility for getting or conveying the message. The teacher's role here is to provide support by praising effective strategies used, and by questioning or reminding to help a child get over or through some difficulties. The child is in control; the teacher assists, as needed, to ensure success. This is akin to a parent assisting through questioning, restating or scaffolding a young child to express more effectively an intended message. Guided reading in the primary grades is replaced by reader response journals in the intermediate grades. Here, teachers provide purposes for which students are to read. Their responses to these assignments are recorded in journals and discussed, individually or in small groups or in whole class groups, with the teacher and/or peers.

Independent reading and writing offer opportunities to establish fluency with the processes, to identify new competencies to be developed, and to establish a sense of control over these processes in accomplishing personally important tasks. Independent reading and writing also offer opportunities to direct one's own learning and to personally evaluate progress by working out problems encountered. Reading dialogue journals and writing folders of work in progress provide vehicles for students in the intermediate grades to work through comprehension and effective written communication with the help of peers and teachers. Through the dialogue journals or conferencing with the teacher and/or peers, students receive suggestions for improving or expanding their communication skills and strategies. Independent reading and writing opportunities may be likened to children's engagement in spoken language exchanges to satisfy personal interests and needs throughout childhood.

IMPAIRED STUDENTS AND THE WHOLE LANGUAGE APPROACH

Historically, poor readers have been immersed in highly repetitive, slow-paced code emphasis experiences. For learning-disabled students, particularly, the view that code mastery is a prerequisite for reading proficiency has prevailed. This has been rooted in the minimal brain dysfunction view of learning disabilities. Many adherents believe that highly structured sound–symbol instruction is the only viable approach to establishing automatic responses to print because of anomalies in the central nervous system. Yet, the validity of these beliefs about both the source of a learning disability and effective instruc-

Independent reading and writing opportunities may be likened to children's engagement in spoken language exchanges to satisfy personal interests and needs throughout childhood.

tional approaches has not been established (Clark, 1988; Coles, 1987). Support for code emphasis programs, and the bottom-up approach in general, is eroding.

A recent review of the best available evidence on the effectiveness of the phonics approach in the general population suggests that systematic phonics is considered to be a weak instructional treatment, producing an early but short-lived advantage, with little potential for affecting the acquisition of literacy (Turner, 1989). Theory and research regarding poor readers is beginning to document that poor readers may have specific difficulty acquiring reading because of more basic difficulties related to language processing (see, for example, Kamhi & Catts, 1989; Vellutino, 1977). Reading problems may be a reflection of language processing problems that specifically impair acquisition of the code via traditional sound–symbol approaches.

Research is also documenting that poor readers begin to fall behind in language skills, specifically in the development of vocabulary (Chall, Jacobs, & Baldwin, 1990) and syntax (Alvermann, 1983), during the intermediate grades. The practice of immersing poor readers in programs designed to boost decoding skills is probably responsible for retarding growth in vocabulary and syntax due to limited exposure to more advanced vocabulary and sentence structure. Poor readers read less, and they read less complex material. To sustain growth in vocabulary and syntax among poor readers, Chall and colleagues (1990) and Alvermann (1983) recommend reading to these children from more complex material than they are capable of reading themselves. The read-to and shared-reading strategies of the whole

language approach appear specifically to address this issue within the context of reading instruction. An emphasis on meaning with a subordinate although critical role for phonological processing (in establishing automatic levels of word recognition), along with consistent attention to growth in vocabulary and syntax in oral and written language, suggest that the whole language approach may be more beneficial for language/reading-impaired students than traditional code-emphasis approaches. This is yet to be substantially documented, however.

Two proponents of a shift away from the current part-to-whole instructional approaches for reading-disabled students are Coles (1987) and Poplin (1988a). Each has presented compelling arguments in favor of approaches that are more holistic and more sensitive to the child's active construction of meaning and world views. In each case, the approach argued is more compatible with the whole language view of teaching and learning than with the traditional view.

Coles calls for abandonment of the view that learning disabilities are caused by conditions inside the child. He proposes that learning disabilities are a consequence of conditions in the environment, including economic, social, instructional, and biological environments. He contends that instructional approaches must take into account the interaction of conditions across these environments as they affect children and as children change as a consequence. One interpretation of this position is that instruction might not only modulate the effects of biological factors, it might actually change, to some extent, the biological support system children apply to learning. Stated another way, instruction that builds on available language and problem-solving abilities might better serve literacy acquisition and, in the process, further enhance the biological structures that undergird all these related abilities.

The whole language philosophy is built on the premise that the development of language, writing, and reading must be understood as interdependent and reciprocal in nature. Poplin (1988a) calls for a shift from the current reductionist paradigm that guides identification and treatment of learning-disabled students through the search for the most fundamental deficit to be overcome. She proposes, instead, a holistic and constructivist view that acknowledges the child's active role in learning and acknowledges that the sum of the bits and pieces of a child's competencies, which we label in a diagnosis, is not as great as the whole package that the child applies in context. Poplin (1988b) proposes that "... the best indicator of what and how someone will learn is what they already know." (p. 405) She maintains that instruction for learning-disabled students should build on what these children know about the contents of the material being taught or the processes to be learned. Teachers should focus on trying to fill in deficit areas. Again, this view is consistent with the whole language view of the process by which literate behavior is acquired.

• • •

Increasingly, research findings regarding language/reading-impaired students and critical reviews of learning theories as they relate to learning-disabled students are converging in the direction of beliefs and practices that currently characterize the whole language philosophy and attendant instructional practices. Students who require direct teaching and repetitive experiences with the fundamental knowledge, skills, and strategies critical for establishing competence in language, writing, and reading, might be better served in an instructional environment that places this direct teaching in the context of meaningful activities, using a whole-to-part frame of reference. However, the critical research base necessary to support such conjecture is yet to be accumulated.

REFERENCES

Alvermann, D. (1983). Reading achievement and linguistic stages: A comparison of disabled readers and Chomsky's 6- to 10-year-olds. *Journal of Research Developments in Education, 16,* 26–31.

Atwell, N. (1987). *In the middle: Writing, reading and learning adolescents.* Portsmouth, N.H.: Heinemann Educational Books.

Bartlett, F.C. (1932). *Remembering: A study in experimental and social psychology.* London, England: Cambridge University Press.

Chall, J. (1968). *Learning to read: The great debate.* New York, N.Y.: McGraw Hill.

Chall, J., Jacobs, V.A., & Baldwin, L.E. (1990). *The reading crisis: Why poor children fall behind.* Cambridge, Mass.: Harvard University Press.

Chomsky, N. (1957). *Syntactic structures.* The Hague, Netherlands: Mouton.

Clark, D. (1988). *Dyslexia: Theory and practice of remedial instruction.* Parkton, Md.: York.

Clark, E.V. (1973). What's in a word? On the child's acquisition of semantics in his first language. In T.E. Moore (Ed.), *Cognitive development and the acquisition of language.* New York, N.Y.: Academic Press.

Coles, G.S. (1987). *The learning mystique: A critical look at "learning disabilities."* New York, N.Y.: Pantheon.

Department of Education. (1985). *Reading in junior*

classes—with guidelines to the revised ready-to-read series. Wellington, New Zealand: Author.

Furth, H.G. (1969). *Piaget and knowledge.* Chicago, Ill.: University of Chicago Press.

Halliday, M.A.K. (1975). *Learning how to mean.* London, England: Edward Arnold.

Holdaway, D. (1979). *Foundations of literacy.* Auckland, New Zealand: Ashton-Scholastic.

Kamhi, A., & Catts, H. (1989). *Reading disabilities: A developmental language perspective.* Boston, Mass.: College Hill Press/Little, Brown.

Kintsch, W., & Van Dijk, T. (1978). Toward a model of text comprehension and production. *Psychological Review, 85,* 363–394.

LaBerge, D., & Samuels, S.J. (1974). Toward a theory of automatic information processing in reading. *Cognitive Psychology, 6,* 293–323.

Michel, P.A. (1990). What first graders think about reading. In R.W. Blake (Ed.), *Whole language: Explorations and applications.* Schenectady, N.Y.: New York State English Council.

Monroe, W.S. (1950). *Teaching-learning theory and teacher education 1890–1950.* New York, N.Y.: Greenwood.

Mooney, M. (1988). *Developing life-long readers.* Wellington, New Zealand: Department of Education.

Mosenthal, P. (1984). Reading comprehension research from a classroom perspective. In J. Flood (Ed.), *Promoting reading comprehension.* Newark, Del.: International Reading Association.

National Assessment of Educational Progress. (1985). *The report card, progress toward excellence in our schools: Trends in reading over for national assessments, 1971–1978.* Princeton, N.J.: National Assessment of Educational Progress.

Perkinson, H.J. (1984). *How we learn from our mistakes.* Westport, Conn.: Greenwood.

Poplin, M.S. (1988a). The reductionist fallacy in learning disabilities: Replicating the past by reducing the present. *Journal of Learning Disabilities, 21,* 389–400.

Poplin, M.S. (1988b). Holistic/constructivist principles of the teaching/learning process: Implications for the field of learning disabilities. *Journal of Learning Disabilities, 21,* 401–416.

Rumelhart, D.E. (1977). Toward an interactive model of reading. In S. Dornic (Ed.), *Attention and performance* (Vol. 6). Hillsdale, N.J.: Erlbaum.

Smith, N.B. (1986). *American reading instruction.* Newark, Del.: International Reading Association.

Snelbecker, G.E. (1974). *Learning theory, instructional theory, and psychoeducational design.* New York, N.Y.: McGraw Hill.

Turner, R.L. (1989). The great debate—can both Carbo and Chall be right? *Phi Delta Kappan, 71,* 276–283.

Vellutino, F.R. (1977). Alternative conceptualizations of dyslexia: Evidence in support of a verbal deficit hypothesis. *Harvard Educational Review, 47* (3), 334–354.

Vygotsky, L.S. (1962). *Thought and language.* (E. Hanfmann & G. Vakar, Eds. and Trans.). Cambridge, Mass.: MIT Press.

Weaver, C. (1988). *Reading process and practice.* Portsmouth, N.H.: Heinemann Educational Books.

Wells, G. (1986). *The meaning makers.* Portsmouth, N.H.: Heinemann Educational Books.

Individual processing in classroom settings

Nickola Wolf Nelson, PhD
Associate Professor
Department of Speech Pathology and
* Audiology*
Western Michigan University
Kalamazoo, Michigan

WHEN CLASSROOM communication expectations exceed the abilities of students, failures occur. When students have difficulties in classrooms, they are often referred for assessment to determine whether they might qualify for special education services. According to federal law (Public Law 94-142), the testing that follows must include more than one assessment device validated for the purpose for which it is used. The assessment requirement is usually interpreted to mean that standardized tests must be administered in a standardized manner. In implementing this procedure, children are typically taken to small, quiet rooms, distractions are minimized, and students work in a one-to-one relationship with an adult.

Michael J. Clark Ph.D., Associate Professor, Western Michigan University, provided helpful suggestions in the preparation of this article. A colleague, Candis Warner's application of family therapy to language intervention with preschool children, motivated the application of system theory to problems of individual processing in classroom contexts.

TLD, 1986, 6(2), 13–27

Similar contextual controls are exerted when scientists seek to understand why children have difficulty learning. They often select subjects who are alike in specified ways. Experimental tasks are then administered, which can be replicated under controlled conditions.

Professionals who perform individual assessment and those engaged in experimental analysis are now rethinking their approaches to studying the ways in which children perform in a variety of settings. Specifically, the wisdom of removing children from naturalistic contexts to learn about their behavior is being questioned. Mishler (1979) refers to research methods based on the traditional application of the scientific method as "context-stripping procedures" (p. 3). He states that "as theorists and researchers, we tend to behave as if context were the enemy of understanding rather than the resource for understanding that it is in our everyday lives" (p. 2).

METHODS OF STUDYING INDIVIDUALS IN CONTEXT

Several methods, drawn from a variety of disciplines, have been suggested for studying individuals in the contexts in which they usually function (Mishler, 1979; van Kleeck, 1985).

Ecological approaches

Ecological approaches are used by psychologists (Bronfenbrenner, 1977; Cole, 1979) and by educational psychologists (Oxford, Morrison, & McKinney, 1979; Schumaker & Deshler, 1984) to study individuals' behavior in a variety of social contexts.

In ecological approaches, even the experimental laboratory is not viewed as context-free, but as a particular type of ecological context with its own contextual effects (Bronfenbrenner, 1977). Similarly, the classroom, the resource room, the home, and the testing room all might be viewed as appropriate ecological contexts for evaluating students' language and learning skills—as long as the unique contributions of each setting are considered in interpreting the observations and findings.

Phenomenological viewpoints

When using ecological approaches to conduct research, a phenomenological view of observational data is assumed. In the phenomenological view, the phenomenon being studied does not have its own objective or "true" characteristics independent of the techniques and methods the observer uses to study it. Rather the phenomenon is intertwined with observer techniques. Since reality contains multiple truths, any of which may appear when the phenomenon is viewed from different perspectives, many equally valid descriptions are possible (Mishler, 1979).

Professionals charged with the responsibility of conducting individual assessments and assisting in goal setting might benefit from using the phenomenological perspective when attempting to reconcile apparently conflicting reports of student behavior by parents, teachers, students, and other evaluators. Rather than assuming that a student has a certain unchanging set of abilities that must be discovered, measured, labeled and treated, the student may be viewed as one participant in a larger system that has its own characteristics. Multiple perspectives can be allowed, since each is accurate in its own right.

System theory

The study of individuals as participants in larger systems is a product of system theory. System theory was conceived by Bertalanffy in Germany during the 1920s as an organismic view of biological systems. He broadened the organismic approach into general systems theory in the 1930s and 1940s (Bertalanffy, 1968). The theory has since been applied widely as a scientific paradigm across many disciplines. System theory is not a discipline in and of itself; rather "it is a meta-discipline whose subject matter can be applied within virtually any other discipline" (Checkland, 1981, p. 5). Bertalanffy describes system theory as a "broad view which far transcends technological problems and demands, a reorientation that has become necessary in science in general and in the gamut of disciplines from physics and biology to the behavioral and social sciences and to philosophy" (Bertalanffy, 1968, p. vii). System theory appears to be ideal for organizing the study of individual processing in classroom settings.

Minuchin (1985) summarizes six basic principles of system theory as they relate

---

System theory appears to be ideal for organizing the study of individual processing in classroom settings.

---

to family therapy. The same principles apply to working with students who have difficulty with the language-processing demands of classrooms.

1. *Any system is an organized whole, and elements within the system are necessarily interdependent.* This is the core concept of system theory. A system approach is the antithesis of "context stripping," as referred to by Mishler (1979). Because individuals are part of systems, they can be understood only in context. For the child who has difficulty in school, system theorists would argue that it would be invalid to seek the reasons for classroom difficulty merely by removing the child from the classroom and testing him or her in isolation. Similarly, treatment approaches that do not involve larger contexts would yield fragmented results. System theory also recognizes that both the teacher and the child are members of other systems, such as family and culture, that must be considered as well.

Furthermore, the child's intrinsic neurological and biological systems are viewed as open systems that interact with external physical events. The brain and its motor and sensory peripherals act as transducers to change extrinsic physical events (e.g., acoustic and light-wave molecular disturbances) into intrinsic physical events (i.e., neurophysiological activity), which are simultaneously experienced as cognitive or linguistic events. The resulting mental activity is not identical for any of the individuals in a classroom, even though it may appear that they have all been exposed to the same set of stimuli.

Also, physical events, such as acoustic signals or printed words on a page, are not viewed as static occurrences with intrinsic, unmodifiable characteristics. Rather, physical events are subject to operations imposed by the individuals who encounter them. Thus a teacher's lecture may be meaningful to one student, may seem like meaningless noise to another, and may seem an unpleasant stimulus to be resisted by a third student.

2. *Patterns in a system are circular rather than linear.* Replacing the notion that one thing causes another, "the model of interaction within a systems point of view involves a spiral of recursive feedback loops" (Minuchin, 1985, p. 290). This model applies both to individual learning systems and to classroom systems. It goes beyond determining which aspects of the classroom curriculum or a language-processing problem (such as attention or auditory memory deficits) might be "causing" the child to have difficulty learning. Rather, a systems orientation recognizes the importance of the interaction among components.

For example, spiral patterns can be used to explain the results of research on children's language comprehension and teachers' classroom discourse. In one study (Nelson, 1976), children 6 to 9 years old were found to perform better on a picture-pointing language comprehension task when sentences were less complex and speaking rate was slower; however, comprehension differences related to speaking rate and sentence difficulty lessened with increased age. In a separate study (Cuda & Nelson, 1976; Nelson, 1984), teachers' speaking rate and sentence complexity were also found to rise significantly from first to sixth grade, but with stair-stepped increases. First- and third-grade teachers both used fewer complex sentences than

sixth-grade teachers, but both third-grade and sixth-grade teachers talked significantly faster than first-grade teachers.

Considering that results from these two studies reflect two aspects of the same system, it makes sense to theorize that, as children's listening rates and syntactic decoding skills gradually increase, teachers' speaking rate and syntactic complexity increase at a similar pace. But which is the cause and which is the effect? According to system theory, each of the elements of the system (in this case, the student and teacher) interacts with the other; therefore, changes occur in the total system over time. Adjustments in physical, structural, and content complexity of academic discourse, both in teacher talk and written textbook language, increase in response to increases in student ability, and also play a role in boosting that ability. However, classrooms are group settings. If discourse demands are geared to the average abilities of children at a certain level, what will be the effect on individual students whose processing resources are out of line with the demands of the system? (See also Silliman, this issue.)

A major responsibility of the evaluation team for such students is to determine how much out of synch they might be. The only way to do so is to consider interactions between and among the student, the classroom, and the additional systems and subsystems in which the student may be involved.

3. *Systems have homeostatic features that maintain the stability of their patterns.* The basic concept of homeostasis is one of maintaining equilibrium and resisting change. The process of maintaining homeostasis is usually "error-activated."

Departures from the expected range of patterns are "controlled, via corrective feedback loops, to reestablish familiar equilibrium" (Minuchin, 1985, p. 290). However, a similar self-regulation process occurs in dysfunctional systems to maintain maladaptive behaviors as familiar and necessary parts of the system.

Speech-language pathologists are familiar with the homeostasis phenomenon as it relates to problems of "carry-over." Although new linguistic skills may be established and demonstrated in an isolated therapy room, when children return to more natural contexts, such as the classroom, they have a strong tendency to return to old patterns of initiating and responding in communicative exchanges. Intervention plans need to include conscious elements designed to reduce the influence of natural resistance to change.

4. *Evolution and change are inherent in open systems.* Although homeostasis is a feature of systems, it is counterbalanced by the companion feature of "morphogenesis" (i.e., change of form) (Minuchin, 1985, p. 290). Morphogenesis is the tendency of systems to respond to disturbances of equilibrium by adapting and eventually developing new patterns of behavior in which equilibrium is restabilized. Adaptation is characteristic of growth and development in all living systems and it is one of Piaget's basic tenets.

The classroom setting presents numerous demands for adaptation. For example, children encounter complexity increments in the language used in classroom settings. Some children adapt to them, but others have difficulty. Understanding the nature of the changes may assist in the remediation of the difficulty.

Another example of adaptation pertains to the transitions children undergo in school. A major characteristic of the transitions from home to classroom, from lower to upper grade levels, and from oral to written language modalities is the increasing decontextualization of language. Home language, compared with school language, and oral language, compared with written language, rely on nonverbal contexts, routines, and familiarity. Cook-Gumperz (1977) uses the term "situated meaning" for communication events that are high in contextual support and describes school and written language contexts as becoming increasingly "lexicalized." Another shift is one in which school language becomes increasingly metalinguistic both as a content subject and the focus of conscious attention (van Kleeck, 1984).

These changes require children to become better at applying linguistic processing strategies to extract meaning from utterances (rather than applying nonlinguistic ones to extract meaning from situations), and at using language to talk about language. Children whose individual processing strategies do not include linguistic decoding and encoding options for complex syntactic structures and semantic relationships experience difficulty as classroom language demands become more complex and nonverbal processing support becomes more meager. When such mismatches are identified (Nelson, 1985; Silliman, 1984), the need for intervention to influence the direction of change in a maladaptive system becomes evident.

The interaction of the tendencies toward homeostasis and morphogenesis implies that "an adaptively reorganized system is not necessarily a more stable system: adaptation is not synonymous with structural stability" (Laszlo, 1972, p. 43). Adaptation of the whole system must be encouraged if changes are to be stabilized. For example, a child may learn in language intervention activities to use a "word stretching" technique for performing phonics activities in which initial or final consonants are identified. If the classroom teacher then consistently reminds the student to use word stretching for doing phonics workbook pages, the stability of the technique as an internalized strategy may be enhanced.

Conversely, the language specialist should be aware of the special "metapragmatic" rules of the classroom (van Kleeck, 1984). Metapragmatic rules are conventions for being called on, taking turns, avoiding talking loudly, staying on topic, asking questions at appropriate times, and other rules for regulating the communicative flow of the classroom. Special intervention activities may help certain students to observe such rules. In other cases, speech-language pathologists and other specialists may be inadvertently at cross-purposes with classroom teachers.

For example, specialists in the special education setting may encourage students to ask questions when they have not understood or have forgotten directions. However, when the students return to their classrooms, teachers may send verbal and nonverbal messages to them such as, *Listen the first time, and then you won't have to ask so many questions!* Which perspective is correct?

A phenomenological view of the system allows both to be "correct." McKinney and Feagans (1983) report from observa-

tions of classroom interactions that learning-disabled children consistently had more interactions with teachers than did other students. A system approach to intervention when question asking is a problem might include (a) working with the teacher to determine to what extent a child's forgetting represents the limits of a language processing system or a behavioral ploy for attention, and (b) helping students develop comprehension, self-verbalization, chunking, and other organizational strategies to become more self-reliant, and then reinforcing those skills when they are used independently. (See also Blank and White, this issue.)

5. *Complex systems are composed of subsystems.* The system of students in classroom settings can be partitioned into subsystems for separate study. For example, the child having difficulty might be viewed as one subsystem. This subsystem functions as it does because of complex interactions of a further subset of neurophysiological, language, learning, and social systems. A primary goal of individual assessment for children who are referred for special services is to describe the various functional systems of the child. Too often, the child is viewed as a closed system, or even a set of several separate closed systems, rather than a subsystem that is an inseparable member of larger, more complex systems.

When children are placed in special classrooms or in a program of intermittent language intervention, it is necessary to consider those elements to be part of a larger system as well. Recent discussions of service delivery models tend to favor classroom contexts for intervention (Fujiki & Brinton, 1984; Lee & Shapero-Fine, 1984;

Simon, 1985). This emphasis on classrooms does not mean that the classroom teacher, in addition to everything else for which he or she is already responsible, must now assume the primary role of language specialist, nor does it mean that the speech-language pathologist should work directly with the child in a corner of the classroom. The implication is one of collaboration. Teacher and specialist should (a) understand each other's roles and how the child functions in multiple contexts, (b) adopt aspects of each other's strategies and materials, and (c) use the same metapragmatic, metacognitive, and metalinguistic forms in instructional sessions with the student.

6. *The subsystems within a larger system are separated by boundaries, and interactions across boundaries are governed by implicit rules and patterns.* As subsystems grow and change, the people within and between them create and maintain patterns that are recurrent and stable (Minuchin, 1985). In providing classroom consultation for children who are having language processing problems, it is critical to consider factors related to boundary maintenance and change.

Some of the boundaries between subsystems are literally and legally recognized and protected. For example, federal law requires that parents provide informed written consent before individual assessment of their children may be initiated. Most building principals require notification whenever an outsider is in the building. The eventual success of classroom consultation for individual students will depend to a certain extent on observing both these boundaries, as well as the less formal, but equally important, ones of the parent and teacher subsystems.

Parents approach individualized education planning meetings with different sets of goals and expectations than professionals and administrators. It is important to help parents define those goals, to respect their validity, and to assist in the process of adapting goals over time.

Teachers also may have varying responses to the notion of applying system theory to resolving the processing problems of students in their classrooms. The boundaries of teachers' self-esteem and their roles as experts in their own classrooms should be respected; if not, boundaries may become barriers.

RECOMMENDATIONS FOR IMPLEMENTATION

Aspects of ecological, phenomenological, and system approaches may be used to guide identification, assessment, and intervention procedures for language-disordered children in the schools. Some recommendations and resources for implementing such strategies are presented here.

Identification

Referral and screening criteria and procedures should be based on behaviors that occur in classrooms. Classroom teachers are in the best position to observe such

> *The boundaries of teachers' self-esteem and their roles as experts in their own classrooms should be respected; if not, boundaries may become barriers.*

behaviors as they occur naturally. Formal and informal inservice training may also help teachers to become more sophisticated observers of individual processing difficulties experienced by students in their classrooms.

Damico and Oller (1980) suggest preparing teachers to use pragmatic indicators to identify students at risk in kindergarten through the fifth grade. The indicators include (a) nonfluent self-expression, (b) unusual delays before responding, (c) nonexplicit and ambiguous vocabulary use, (d) irrelevant responses, and (e) poor topic maintenance. Boyce and Larson (1983) and McKinley and Lord-Larson (1985) have developed a procedure that invites teachers to use a five-point interval scale to rate multiple aspects of (a) cognition, (b) language comprehension and listening skills, (c) language production and conversational skills, and (d) survival language. Myklebust's (1971) "Pupil Rating Scale" is another tool designed to facilitate a teacher's observational comments in a variety of subsystem areas.

Parents and students should also be viewed as important members of the identification system. For example, Boyce and Larson (1983) and Lee and Shapero-Fine (1984) suggest providing opportunities for secondary students to refer themselves for special education assessment.

Assessment

Individual assessment based on system theory involves more than administering a few standardized tests and writing up their results. Although a system theory approach is generally more time consuming than traditional assessment, it allows for considerable latitude in the manner of data collection. In addition to using one or more of the rating scales listed above, open-ended interviews with parents, teachers, and students provide multiple perspectives on the system being studied.

Areas to be covered with *parents* are (a) early development, (b) medical history (especially middle ear problems), (c) educational history, (d) anecdotal evidence of specific problems within the past year or so, (e) a review of the problems the parents view as most critical, and (f) their goals for their child's future.

Interviews with *teachers* should collect (a) objective information about the child's academic performance in a variety of subject areas, from both achievement test results and classroom records, (b) descriptions of the child's classroom strengths, (c) a review of the problems the teacher identifies as being most important, (d) anecdotal descriptions of recent classroom events with which the child has experienced difficulty, (e) the teacher's estimate of which aspects of the curriculum present the greatest difficulties for the child, and (f) the teacher's view of the child's learning potential within the current school year and in the future.

Students should be asked for (a) their descriptions of what is hardest about school, (b) their descriptions of what they like best about school, (c) anecdotal accounts of recent classroom events that made them feel really good, (d) anecdotal accounts of recent classroom events that made them feel really bad, and (e) their ideas about what they would like to do as they get older.

A system-based assessment also includes direct and indirect (tape recorded) obser-

| | Comprehensive Assessment of Individuals | | |
Rule systems	Modalities	Linguistic levels	Contexts
Phonological	Listening	Sound	Formal Tests
Morphological	Speaking	Syllable	Spontaneous Samples
Syntactic	Reading	Word	Academic Materials
Semantic	Writing	Sentence	• Workbook Pages
Pragmatic	Thinking°	Complex Sentence	• Reading Text
		Text	• Grade Level
			• Reading Level
			• Science Text
			• Problem Solving

°"Thinking language" is observed as verbal mediation ability. The ability to consciously "talk through" an academic task, or classroom routine, represents metacognitive, metapragmatic, and metalinguistic skill (depending on the task), and is an important part of the individualized assessment of a student having difficulty in classroom contexts.

vation of classroom interactions and a review of curricular materials. More or less formal analyses of teacher and textbook language can also be performed. The findings from such analyses may be related to the child's abilities, measured with formal and informal assessment procedures. A number of resources are available to assist in the analysis of teacher and textbook language (Boyce & Larson, 1983; Gruenewald & Pollack, 1984; Nelson, 1984, 1985; Silliman, 1984; Simon, 1985; Vetter, 1982). Calfee and Sutter (1982) also suggest setting up a special diagnostic discussion session between a teacher and a small group of students that includes the target student. The language specialist observes and takes notes, makes an audio recording, and holds postdiscussion interviews with both the teacher and the student to check perceptions and give feedback.

A system approach does not rule out the possibility of using traditional assessment tools to identify specific abilities and individual problem areas in controlled condi-

tions. Such procedures should not be used exclusively, however, and caution is required in the interpretation of findings.

The comprehensive assessment should include (a) observation of the student's ability to use phonological, morphological, syntactic, semantic, and pragmatic rule systems in a variety of linguistic contexts (at sound, word, sentence, and text levels), and in all language modalities (listening, speaking, reading, and writing); (b) a variety of stimulus materials, including some formal tests or subtests with highly controlled stimuli, and some less formal materials sampled from the classroom environment; and (c) observation of the student's related performance skills, including the ability to focus and maintain attention and to organize information for recall in multiple contexts (see boxed material).

An integrated assessment was made of a third-grade student with a history of speech and language delay. This student was not placed in special education although she was failing all tests on newly introduced content subjects in science and social studies. Her difficulty was analyzed by observing her approach to answering the study questions at the end of a textbook chapter. One of them was an "occasional question" requiring the student to fill in a blank (Mallinson, Mallinson, Brown, Knapp, & Smallwood, 1978, p. 70):

To measure _____ , multiply the distance something moves by the force needed to move it.

To answer this question correctly, it was necessary to return to the paragraph in the text in which the key words of the study sentence occurred (p. 162):

In the upper grades you will learn more about measuring work. For now, just remember that work is measured by multiplying two things. These are the distance an object moves multiplied by the force needed to move it.

It soon became apparent that the student was not able to identify the synonymy of these two passages, and was unable to use linguistic strategies to find the answer. This problem also led to difficulty transforming syntactic structures to perform reciprocal defining and labeling functions. For example, she was able (with a little practice) to fill in the blank in the definition, A machine made up of several different simple machines is called a _____ (complex machine)," but she was unable to complete the following sentence: A complex machine is made up of several _____ (simple machines). These two sentences seemed to her to be entirely different, rather than merely having different surface structures and sharing the same deep structure.

Another problem that became apparent

when the science text was used concerned her difficulty integrating linguistic and cognitive processing strategies to organize information into superordinate, subordinate, and coordinate classes. For example, she was able to list the five kinds of simple machines (lever, wedge, pulley, inclined plane, and wheel-and-axle) but, in response to a question regarding what part of a lever is hinged, she responded "wheel-and-axle." Because she had not used classification strategies to analyze "wheel-and-axle" as being an example of the superordinate category "simple machines," on the same level as "levers," "wheel-and-axle" became eligible to be a subset of "levers."

Feuerstein (1979) has developed a strategy for performing the informal type of observational procedure described above in a more formalized manner. What he terms the Learning Potential Assessment Device (LPAD) is actually a model "upon which a great variety of assessment tools can be constructed" (p. 92). Using this type of procedure, a subject is given a problem, task, or situation to solve that might be (a) logicoverbal, (b) numerical, (c) spatial, (d) pictorial-concrete, (e) figural, or (f) verbal in nature. The solution to the problem entails the use of a cognitive processing strategy such as analogy, seriation, logical multiplication, permutation, syllogism, or classification. The subject is first given the training necessary to solve the initial problem and is then observed in situations that represent more complex versions of the original training task.

Observation of how the student learns when the assessment process includes instruction is an important part of conducting a complete assessment of the whole system. In addition, system views, such as those of Feuerstein (1979), deny that such abilities as "intelligence" are static, unchanging systems. Rather, abilities are seen as malleable subsystems that can change with intervention.

Intervention

A system approach to intervention is a natural outgrowth of the assessment process. In fact, the blending of assessment and intervention activities (as, for example, in Feuerstein's method) is characteristic of classroom consultation, and is an example of reciprocal interaction within systems.

Four principles of intervention derive from a systems approach. The first principle is that the activities of intervention should approximate those of "real-life" contexts and should be as intact as possible. The degree of complexity, however, should be controlled so that the student can achieve greater success than he or she would in the truly "natural" environment. For example, the third-grade student described above might be given a series of definition problems in a row, rather than being asked to perform tasks involving a mixture of linguistic structures, as a text might present them. Gradually, the different types of structures could be mixed.

Tyack (1981) reports on a strategy for teaching comprehension of complex sentences to a fifth-grade child who had difficulty with reading comprehension and who had been described as having "some auditory disturbances" and "difficulties in the auditory area" (Tyack, 1981, p. 50). Rather than working on auditory

perceptual skills, Tyack found it more useful to work directly on the linguistic skills that would help the student understand what she read and heard. The student did this by identifying the specific types of complex sentences she did not understand. The identification was made using a variety of contexts, including (a) spontaneous speech, (b) reading and paraphrasing sentences from grade level texts, and (c) responding to specially designed pretest sentence sets (e.g., "George is the only boy in this class who has ever been to France"; "Who has been to France?") (Tyack, 1981, p. 51). Then intervention sequences were designed to teach production and comprehension of each of the complex sentence types on which more than two errors occurred on the 20-item pretest.

The intervention sequences were designed using a step-by-step approach, written language stimuli, and metalinguistic focus on the meaning and relationships of the underlying simple sentences. For example, a six-step sequence was used to teach coordinated sentences with the subject deleted in the second sentence. Among the intervention steps were those for the student (a) to mark "S" next to the subjects of typewritten sentence pairs (Sam [S] found a cat. Sam [S] took it home); (b) to draw a line through the coreferential subject in the second sentence (Sam found a cat and ~~Sam~~ took it home); and (c) to produce or to paraphrase the complex sentence type.

At the end of the six months intervention program the student completed programs on 11 different complex sentence types, plus additional work on *Wh*-question forms, pronoun reference, other anaphoric references, and synonymous and antonymous word meanings, Tyack's (1981) student had made remarkable progress as measured by spontaneous communication and classroom tasks in listening, speaking, reading, and writing. Tyack's program is a quintessential example of an intervention program that achieves a balance between keeping learning tasks intact, and yet presenting them to the student in units small enough that learning can take place.

A second principle of intervention is that its linguistic objectives should be comprehensive in scope. Information from assessment about the student's difficulties with the content, form, and use of language in a variety of modalities and in a variety of contexts should guide the selection of intervention targets. For the most part, strong areas can be used to facilitate weak ones. If the student has learned to overuse some linguistic systems at the expense of others, tasks should be designed with increasing complexity that reduce the student's dependence on the stronger skills and require the use of the weaker skills. For example, a student who, during oral reading, omits function words or misreads them, may need practice (a) identifying function words apart from their sentence contexts (e.g., from drill cards); (b) reading and acting out different sentences that have the same content words, but different function words; and, eventually, (c) reading and paraphrasing a classroom text, perhaps all in the same session.

A third principle is that school-age students who need intervention for classroom difficulties should be taught strategies rather than academic content (McKinley & Lord-Larson, 1985). One method for achieving this goal is to develop knowledge and performance strategies for the phonologic, morphologic, semantic, syntactic, and pragmatic systems and bring these systems to the meta-level of consciousness (see, for example, Alley & Deshler, 1979; Deshler, Warner, Schumaker, & Alley, 1983; Schumaker & Deshler, 1984; Schumaker, Deshler, Alley, Warner, & Denton, 1982; Schwartz & McKinley, 1984; Wong & Jones, 1982).

The procedures advocated by Feuerstein (1979) also provide a model for system-oriented intervention that can be applied in a variety of spheres. In Feuerstein's system, mediated learning experience is used. Mediated learning experience is defined as those interactional processes by which an experienced adult interposes himself or herself between the developing child and ongoing events through framing, selecting, focusing, and feeding back experience (Feuerstein, 1979). The purpose of mediating experience is to internalize within the child strategies for obtaining and interpreting information.

One type of task Feuerstein uses to accomplish this internalizing process consists of verbal analogies. Verbal analogies are used after the student has learned to engage in self-mediation on nonverbal analogy tasks. An example of Feuerstein's (1979, p. 365) verbal analogies appears in Figure 1. Using this problem, Feuerstein would (a) have students provide a short sentence that connects the two words, "fur coat" and "winter," (b) remind them that the same relationship that exists in the row above must be found in the row below, (c) have them select the word that should be in the lower right frame by using it in a

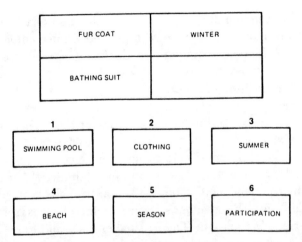

Figure 1. Sample problem from Feurstein's (1979, p. 365) Analogies Test. Reprinted with the permission of Scott, Foresman, Glenview, Illinois.

sentence that is like the one they used for the top row, and (d) discuss why each of the choices not selected was not as good as the one that was chosen. For example, "swimming pool" is not correct because the question is *when* you wear a bathing suit and not where you wear it; "clothing" is not correct because it tells what a bathing suit is and not when it is worn; number 3 is the correct answer because it is the specific season, just as winter is a specific season; and so forth. Over a series of problems of this sort, students learn the strategy of self-questioning to arrive at the correct solution. Thus, the "thinking language" (the author's term) the child acquires during intervention becomes part of a comparing and contrasting strategy that can be applied to solve a wide variety of academic problems.

A fourth principle is that intervention should represent comprehensive efforts to integrate the various subsystems involved, both human and physical. The goals and priorities of students, teachers, parents, speech-language pathologists, and other

> *The goals and priorities of students, teachers, parents, speech-language pathologists, and other specialists must all be honestly considered in establishing intervention objectives.*

specialists must all be honestly considered in establishing intervention objectives.

It is also important that individuals in the system be given information about the process of change so that they can become agents of positive change. For example, teachers can be given information in preservice and inservice settings about general ways in which they can foster a better match between their talking and their students' listening (Nelson, 1985). When individual students in their classrooms are identified as having difficulty, ongoing communication can help all those who work with the child coordinate their efforts in more specific ways. For example, they might modify the metalanguage they use with the child in order to reduce confusion when the child moves among learning settings.

In addition, intervention planners should consider physical subsystems, such as classroom acoustics, to be continuous with psychological and linguistic subsystems. For example, if the child appears to be adversely affected by noise, the classroom's acoustic environment could be improved by amplifying the teacher's speech or by sound-treating the room. The child's ability to focus on the teacher's message in the presence of competing noise can be increased by introducing competing auditory signals (perhaps from taped television commercials) during individual language intervention sessions).

•　•　•

None of the procedures described here should be viewed as particularly mysterious or special. They do not require unique training. What they do require is the ability of all involved to be able to shift their points of focus from larger systems to smaller ones, and to be able to partition a problem so that it becomes more manageable without losing sight of the system as a whole.

REFERENCES

Alley, G.R., & Deshler, D.D. (1979). *Teaching the learning disabled adolescent: Strategies and methods.* Denver, CO: Love Publishing Co.

Bertalanffy, L. von (1968). *General system theory.* New York: George Braziller.

Bronfenbrenner, U. (1977). Toward an experimental ecology of human development. *American Psychologist, 32,* 513–531.

Boyce, N.L., & Larson, V.L. (1983). *Adolescents' communication: Development and disorders.* Eau Claire, WI: Thinking Ink Publications.

Calfee, R., & Sutter, L. (1982). Oral language assessment through formal discussion. *Topics in Language Disorders, 2*(4), 20–33.

Checkland, P. (1981). *Systems thinking, systems practice.* Chichester, England: Wiley & Sons.

Cole, M. (1979). Foreword. In U. Bronfenbrenner (Ed.), *The ecology of human development.* Cambridge, MA: Harvard University Press.

Cook-Gumperz, J. (1977). Situated instructions: Language socialization of schoolage children. In S. Ervin-Tripp and C. Mitchell-Kernan (Eds.), *Child discourse.* New York: Academic Press.

Cuda, R.A., & Nelson, N.W. (1976, November). *Analysis of teacher speaking rate, syntactic complexity and hesitation phenomena as a function of grade level.* Paper presented at the meeting of the American Speech-Language-Hearing Association, Houston, TX.

Damico, J., & Oller, J.W., Jr. (1980). Pragmatic versus morphological/syntactic criteria for language referrals. *Language, Speech, and Hearing Services in Schools, 11,* 85–94.

Deshler, D.D., Warner, M.M., Schumaker, J.B., & Alley, G.R. (1983). Learning strategies intervention model: Key components and current status. In J. McKinney & L. Feagans (Eds.), *Current topics in learning disabilities* (Vol. 1). Norwood, NJ: Ablex.

Feuerstein, R. (1979). *The dynamic assessment of retarded performers.* Baltimore, MD: University Park Press.

Fujiki, M., & Brinton, B. (1984). Supplementing language therapy: Working with the classroom teacher. *Language, Speech, and Hearing Services in Schools, 15,* 98–109.

Gruenewald, L.J., & Pollack, S.A. (1984). *Language interaction in teaching and learning.* Baltimore, MD: University Park Press.

Laszlo, E. (1972). *Introduction to systems philosophy.* New York: Gordon and Breach, Science Publishers.

Lee, A.D., & Shapero-Fine, J. (1984). In G.P. Wallach & K.G. Butler (Eds.), *Language learning disabilities in school-age children* (pp. 338–359). Baltimore, MD: Williams & Wilkins.

Mallinson, G.G., Mallinson, J.B., Brown, D.G., Knapp, J., Jr., & Smallwood, W.L. (1978). *Science: Understanding your environment.* Morristown, NJ: Silver Burdett Co.

McKinley, N.L., & Lord-Larson, V. (1985). Neglected language-disordered adolescent: A delivery model.

Language, Speech, and Hearing Services in Schools, 16, 2–15.

McKinney, J.D., & Feagans, L. (1983). Adaptive classroom behavior of learning disabled students. *Annual Review of Learning Disabilities, 1,* 72–79.

Minuchin, P. (1985). Families and individual development: Provocations from the field of family therapy. *Child Development, 56,* 289–302.

Mishler, E.G. (1979). Meaning in context: Is there any other kind? *Harvard Educational Review, 49,* 1–19.

Myklebust, H.R. (1971). *The pupil rating scale: Screening for learning disabilities.* New York: Grune & Stratton.

Nelson, N.W. (1976). Comprehension of spoken language by normal children as a function of speaking rate, sentence difficulty, and listener age and sex. *Child Development, 47,* 299–303.

Nelson, N.W. (1984). Beyond information processing: The language of teachers and textbooks. In G.P. Wallach & K.G. Butler (Eds.), *Language learning disabilities in school-age children* (pp. 154–178). Baltimore, MD: Williams & Wilkins.

Nelson, N.W. (1985). Teacher talk and child listening—Fostering a better match. In C. Simon (Ed.), *Communication and classroom skills in school-aged children: Assessment and programming methodologies* (pp. 65–96). San Diego, CA: College-Hill Press.

Oxford, R.B., Morrison, S.B., & McKinney, J.D. (1979). Classroom ecology and off-task behavior on kindergarten students. *Journal of Classroom Interaction, 15,* 34–40.

Schumaker, J.B., & Deshler, D.D. (1984). Setting demand variables. *Topics in Language Disorders, 4*(2), 22–40.

Schumaker, J.B., Deshler, D.D., Alley, G.R., Warner, M.M., & Denton, P.H. (1982). Multipass: A learning strategy for improving reading comprehension. *Learning Disability Quarterly, 5,* 295–304.

Schwartz, L., & McKinley, N.L. (1984). *Daily communication: Strategies for the language disordered adolescent.* Eau Claire, WI: Thinking Ink Publications.

Silliman, E.R. (1984). Interactional competencies in the instructional context: The role of teaching discourse in learning. In G.P. Wallach & K.G. Butler (Eds.), *Language learning disabilities in school-age children* (pp. 288–317). Baltimore, MD: Williams & Wilkins.

Simon, C.S. (Ed.). (1985). *Communication skills and classroom success: Therapy methodologies for language-learning disabled students.* San Diego, CA: College-Hill Press.

Tyack, D.L. (1981). Teaching complex sentences. *Language, Speech, and Hearing Services in Schools, 12,* 49–56.

van Kleeck, A. (1984). Metalinguistic skills: Cutting across spoken and written language and problem-solving abilities. In G.P. Wallach & K.G. Butler (Eds.), *Language learning disabilities in school-age children* (pp. 128–153). Baltimore, MD: Williams & Wilkins.

van Kleeck, A. (1985). Issues in adult—child interaction: six philosophical orientations. *Topics in Language Disorders, 5*(2), 1–15.

Vetter, D.K. (1982). Language disorders and schooling. *Topics in Language Disorders, 2*(4), 13–19.

Wong, B.Y.L., & Jones, W. (1982). Increasing metacomprehension in learning disabled and normally achieving students through self-questioning training. *Learning Disability Quarterly, 5,* 228–240.

Questions: A powerful but misused form of classroom exchange

Marion Blank, PhD
Children's Hearing Institute
Manhattan Eye & Ear Hospital
New York, New York

Sheila J. White, PhD
Research Department
Lexington Center for the Hearing
Impaired
Jackson Heights, New York

THE EXCHANGE that follows (Peshkin, 1978, p. 102) is unique yet familiar:

Teacher: OK, current events, Glenn?
Student: Pablo Casals, the well-known cellist, died at ninety-six.
Teacher: Ok, shush! Jim?
Student: The war over in the Middle East is still going on.
Teacher: Is it going on in the same way? Frank?
Student: Egypt asked for Syria to intervene. They want a security meeting or a quick meeting of the U.N. Security Council.
Teacher: Ok, for what reason? Do you know? Anyone know why Egypt called a meeting of the Security Council of the U.N.? What has the Security Council just initiated?
Student: A cease-fire.

The passage bears the unmistakable stamp of the classroom. This type of exchange takes place in few other contexts. At the same time, few other types of exchange take place at school. Because of the power-

TLD, 1986, 6(2), 1–12
© 1986 Aspen Publishers, Inc.

ful role that school plays in the U.S. culture, its unique form of classroom dialogue has come under increasing scrutiny (e.g., Bloom, 1976; Flanders, 1970).

This examination has led to criticism of school language on the basis of its uniqueness. In this view, because school language contains patterns of exchange that are unfamiliar to children, it is a source of confusion and failure. Critics of school language also claim that children may not be exposed to its forms in any other situation. However, many situations are accompanied by unique linguistic patterns. For example, a physician, unlike other members of our society, is allowed to say, "Please take off your clothes" to a perfect stranger. Obviously, no one would suggest that the privilege be withdrawn on the grounds that it represents unique language.

Rather than uniqueness, a central issue concerning school language is whether the language of the classroom is consistent with the school's objectives. While schools have multiple goals, clearly a primary objective is to enhance thinking and cognition (e.g., Stevenson, Parker, Wilkinson, Bonnevaux, & Gonzalez, 1978). Language is essential to this objective since it is the major symbolic system that human beings use to guide their thoughts and ideas. The central concern of this article is to what extent does the form of classroom dialogue meet the stated objectives of the school.

In approaching this issue, emphasis will be given to questions, since of all the components of classroom exchange, questioning plays a dominant role. In the opening example, the adult has the prerogative for posing questions, and exercises it often.

Every one of the teacher's turns contains at least one question. The prevalence of question asking on the part of the teaching adult is one of the characteristics that makes school dialogue so readily identifiable. Indeed, teachers use questions nearly exclusively to carry out their objectives for educating children.

Many investigators have examined the role of questions in classroom dialogue and found definite patterns. An overriding pattern is a three-part sequence consisting of question, answer, and acknowledgment (Bellack, Kliebard, Hyman, & Smith, 1966; Mishler, 1978). The numerous critiques of the question mode that have followed this research have been based on the premise that (a) questions do not allow a free exchange of ideas, (b) they are formulated in such a way that the children must produce a narrow, predetermined set of responses, and (c) when asked by a questioner who knows the answers, basic pragmatic rules are violated. (See Dillon, 1982a, 1982b, for an extensive review of these issues.)

The problems associated with an overreliance on questions are, in fact, far more profound than even many current critiques would suggest. The question form is clearly an invaluable component of verbal exchange. However, it has been made to carry a responsibility that no single linguistic form could possibly bear without becoming massively distorted. Such distortion is indeed what has taken place. Ironically, because the distortion is ubiquitous, it has taken on a degree of familiarity that permits it to go unnoticed.

In an effort to highlight some of these problems, this article will examine four question-asking practices that prevail in schools. Two of them stem from the goal of fostering cognitive development. These are: (1) maximizing the number of high-level questions asked, and (2) translating a student's lack of knowledge into questions. The other two derive from certain aspects of social skills that have generally received little conscious attention. Each will be discussed in turn.

MAXIMIZING HIGHER LEVEL QUESTIONS

Given that a primary goal of asking questions is to stimulate thought, teachers are often urged to improve the quality of their questions. This suggestion appears in many forms: that divergent rather than convergent questions be used; that open-ended rather than closed-ended questions be asked, queries demand reasons rather than facts, and that they stimulate thought rather than evoke rote memory (Bloom, 1976; Flanders, 1970; Pressley & Forrest-Pressley, 1985). The focus on higher-level questions has an intuitive appeal. It is consistent with the respected Socratic method by which thought-provoking questions lead a student to knowledge. Simple questions are thought to have no such power and thus are assumed to be counterproductive to intellectual goals.

Yet the injunction to use higher-level

Given that a primary goal of asking questions is to stimulate thought, teachers are often urged to improve the quality of their questions.

---

questions carries with it the assumption that the child can comprehend the question that is asked. The fact that *questions themselves carry a cognitive load*, which is especially great in higher-order questions, is largely overlooked. An example can serve to illustrate the point. A study was conducted (Blank, 1975) to determine the reasoning processes children used in a learning task. When 3-year-olds were asked *why* they made the choices they did, they responded in the "egocentric" style that Piaget had identified in children of that age. When the question was changed to the simpler form, *Which ones* (referring to the stimuli) *were right?*, the children's responses were accurate and focused. Clearly, the children's knowledge had not changed; instead, their access to this knowledge varied according to the type and level of complexity of the question asked (Blank, 1975).

When a child's limitations are obvious, the importance of question complexity is accorded the consideration it merits—even though it is not explicitly acknowledged. For example, an adult might well ask a toddler, *Where is your nose?*, but would not conceive of asking *Why do we need noses?* in the belief that higher-order questions are an absolute good. With children who are capable of extended verbal formulations, however, such judgments are more difficult. The fact that children are capable of producing a flow of words often leads to the incorrect assumption that they are ready for any and all questions. Not only is this assumption false, but it can also have particularly tragic consequences for learning-disabled children. It makes children who are already uncertain experience the additional pain of shame and failure.

The following segment of dialogue illustrates this phenomenon. The child in the dialogue has been diagnosed as having difficulties in problem solving and causal reasoning. In an effort to stimulate these functions, the teacher, using a poster depicting a jungle being consumed by fire, seeks to help the child recognize the cause of the fire:

Teacher: How could grass in a jungle get on fire?

Child: 'Cause they (*referring to animals*) have to stay in the jungle.

Teacher: (*in an incredulous tone*) You mean the grass gets on fire because the animals stay in the jungle?

Child: Yeah.

Teacher: I don't think so. What if there was a fire in somebody's house—

Child: (*interrupting*) Then they're dead, or hurt.

Teacher: Yeah, they'd be hurt. But how would a fire start in somebody's house?

Child: By starting something with matches.

Teacher: A match, okay. Now do you think this fire could have started with a match?

Child: Yeah.

Teacher: This fire in the jungle? Who would have a match in the jungle? The animals?

Child: A monkey.

Teacher: A monkey would have a match in the jungle?

Child: (*nodding*) I saw that on TV. . . .

The discussion about the fire continued for another 17 exchanges, at which point it was abandoned because the teacher saw no way to move the child beyond the confusion he or she was experiencing.

This example of the failure brought about by higher-level questioning is by no means unique. Extensive data demonstrate the futility of this approach, particularly with learning-disabled children (Blank, Rose, & Berlin, 1978a; Parnell, Patterson, & Harding, 1984). One path for avoiding this problem is offered by the model proposed by Blank, Rose, and Berlin (1978a, 1978b), in which language formulations, including questions, vary along a continuum of abstraction. That is, language is seen as varying in closeness to or distance from concrete perceptual experience. For example, the *perceptual-verbal distance* is greater when children are asked to assess the similarity between two things (*How are* X *and* Y *alike?*) than when they are asked to label them (*What are they called?*). The recognition of a question's complexity in terms of its perceptual-verbal distance is a first step toward minimizing the likelihood of failure. The second step is to assess a child prior to instruction and then design the exchange specifically for the child's level, rather than asking questions that would almost certainly provoke failure.

In the case of a child who cannot answer causal questions, as in the jungle dialogue, these questions can be avoided and precursors to this skill can be tapped. For example, the teacher could have the child focus on available material by asking simpler questions such as *What is happening?* or *What are the animals doing?* There are also other methods available to move children beyond the level at which they are functioning. The next section considers some of these methods.

TRANSLATING IDENTIFIED WEAKNESS INTO QUESTIONS

In the jungle dialogue, questions about the cause of the fire were asked not only because they were "higher level," but also because they represented spheres in which the child had been shown to display clear deficiencies (i.e., diagnostic testing had shown causal thinking to be an area of weakness for this child). The step from diagnosis to treatment was to translate the identified weakness into a question *that required the child to use the very skill that he or she had been shown to lack.*

Educators have, of course, long debated whether to teach to a child's strengths or weaknesses. To the extent that the strategy of "teaching to weakness" is adopted, it is commonly implemented by asking the child questions in the area of identified deficiencies. In the jungle fire example, the questions also happened to coincide with what had been considered as higher-level questions for a preschool-age child. However, the translation of deficiencies into questions exists at all levels of cognitive complexity. Thus a child who has been shown not to know colors is repeatedly asked to identify colors; one who has been shown not to know numbers is asked questions about numbers; and one who has been shown not to understand spatial and directional concepts is asked questions involving prepositions (*under, over, near,* etc.).

The obvious outcome of this practice is that the classroom becomes a setting in which children do not overcome their difficulties, but instead must confront them continually in the form of questions that are bound to lead to failure. Dealing with this problem does not necessarily involve avoiding the failure, but rather developing techniques that will allow children to handle it. Essentially, a process of simplification is required that is related to a continuum of abstraction (Blank, Rose, Berlin, 1978a, 1978b). Specifically, when children fail because questions are beyond their level of information or skill, the teaching adult should reformulate the problem at a simpler level. The following dialogue illustrates a simplification sequence:

Adult: Why do we use tape for hanging pictures?
Child: 'Cause it's shiny.
Adult: Here's a shiny piece of paper and here's a shiny piece of tape. Let's try them both. Try hanging the picture with the shiny paper.
Child: (*does it*)
Adult: Does it work?
Child: No, it's falling.
Adult: Now, try the tape.
Child: (*does it*)
Adult: Does it work?
Child: Yeah, its not falling.
Adult: So, why do we use the tape for hanging pictures?
Child: It won't fall.

In this sequence, the teacher had posed a *why*-question to which the child offered an incorrect response. The teacher then reduced the level of the demand. After the intermediate steps were dealt with adequately, the original question was repeated and was answered correctly. Thus the simplification sequence involves a carefully controlled dialogue that leads the child to appropriate responses. Furthermore, the sequence is structured so that the child is helped to see how ideas are connected and subordinated to each other.

RETHINKING COGNITION

Even though the practices of maximizing higher-level questions and focusing on weaknesses may be counter-productive, nevertheless, questions are products of explicit thinking about school language. Rightly or wrongly, these strategies did not develop by chance. Rather they represented conscious efforts to foster cognition. It was thought that children would be helped to expand their intellectual world by being asked to think and talk about physical phenomena. The question-asking strategies that follow from this approach fit comfortably with longstanding societal views about cognition. Piaget's preeminent theory, which stresses the concepts of time, space, and causality, clearly represents this view of "cognition." Knowledge related to the physical world is so central in our culture that the term *cognition* has become almost synonymous with conceptual-symbolic functions.

The exclusion of other types of knowledge from the term cognition has become apparent in recent years with studies of what has come to be known as *social cognition* (Hoffman, 1981; Shantz, 1975; Turiel, 1978). The qualifying term *social* has been inserted to acknowledge the fact that a person's ability to cooperate with other members of the human community also involves cognitive skills, albeit ones that may operate under quite different rules from those in the conceptual-symbolic realm. This recognition represents a major advance in psychological research. No longer will a single term suffice to represent the broad range of skills involved in effective human functioning. Rather, at a minimum, two domains must be distinguished. In line with currently developing terminology (e.g., Hoffman, 1981), *nonsocial cognition* will be used here to refer to what has traditionally been termed cognition (i.e., the skills, such as those Piaget described, that underlie humans' understanding of the physical world). *Social cognition* will refer to the skills underlying effective human interaction (Shantz, 1975).

The two sets of skills underlie verbal communication as well; cognition concerns the role of language in conceptual and logical thinking (particularly as it relates to the physical world), while social cognition concerns the role of language in dealing with other people (e.g., indicating feelings, intentions, and moods). Joint consideration of the two domains is essential in order to recognize the intricate social and conceptual underpinnings of each and every utterance.

The recognition of this distinction has important implications for school language. While the goals of the school have led teachers to concentrate on the nonsocial aspects of language, as with any situation involving interacting human beings, the social component is powerful and omnipresent. Because of its lack of recognition, however, teachers have often accommodated to it by using unconscious modes that often operate in counter-productive ways. The role of social factors in questioning is, if anything, more significant and more deeply ingrained than the nonsocial factors discussed earlier. However, social techniques have not developed from conscious analysis of the problems they address. Rather, as in so much of our social functioning, they represent unconscious modes of adapting to intricate, unstated demands of maintaining social interactions when untenable constraints have been imposed.

The material that follows will evaluate two questioning strategies that reflect important social components in the teacher–child exchange. They are using questions to create a shared context and using questions to avoid explicitly criticizing the child.

Using questions to create a shared context

No discussion can take place unless the participants enter a particular form of social contract; namely, they must understand and accept the notion that a particular topic will be pursued in a sustained manner. In this intricate process, participants make ongoing accommodations whereby misunderstandings are dealt with immediately so that the conversation may proceed productively. A variety of strategies, both verbal and nonverbal, are used to achieve accommodation. For example, confusion may be signalled nonverbally through a facial expression or verbally through the use of a statement such as, *What did you just say? I didn't understand it.* Regardless of the form, the aim clearly is to establish and maintain a mutual frame of reference.

The process of creating a shared context takes a quite different form in the classroom. An example of the school-grounded process can be seen in the initial lines of the current events dialogue presented earlier (Peshkin, 1978, p. 102):

Teacher: OK, current events. Glenn?
Student: Pablo Casals, the well-known cellist, died at ninety-six.
Teacher: OK, shush! Jim?
Student: The war over in the Middle East is still going on.
Teacher: Is it going on in the same way? Frank?

In the first utterance, the teacher attempts to establish the topic in a clear, though terse, manner. Its development, however, takes a rather peculiar form. The teacher's second utterance is markedly different from the third utterance, even though both utterances are responses to well-meaning and well-formulated statements on the part of the two students. Although it is not made explicit, it is evident that the teacher's response to Jim is one of acceptance while the response to Glenn is one of nonacceptance.

The differential acceptance, in turn, implies that there is more to the teacher's question than "meets the ear." The teacher asks for a discussion on current events, with no qualification added to the term. Nevertheless, the teacher's responses indicate that what is wanted is information concentrating on the latest international conflict, which is a highly qualified subset of current events. This is not stated, however, in the opening question or in the modes that often operate in counter-productive ways. The role of social factors in questioning is, if anything, more significant and more deeply ingrained than the nonsocial factors discussed earlier. However, social techniques have not developed from conscious analysis of the problems they address. Rather, as in so much of our social functioning, they represent unconscious modes of adapting to intricate, unstated demands of maintaining social interactions when untenable constraints have been imposed.

The material that follows will evaluate two questioning strategies that reflect important social components in the teacher–child exchange. They are using questions to create a shared context and using questions to avoid explicitly criticizing the child.

Using questions to create a shared context

No discussion can take place unless the participants enter a particular form of social contract; namely, they must understand and accept the notion that a particular topic will be pursued in a sustained manner. In this intricate process, participants make ongoing accommodations whereby misunderstandings are dealt with immediately so that the conversation may proceed productively. A variety of strategies, both verbal and nonverbal, are used to achieve accommodation. For example, confusion may be signalled nonverbally through a facial expression or verbally through the use of a statement such as, *What did you just say? I didn't understand it.* Regardless of the form, the aim clearly is to establish and maintain a mutual frame of reference.

The process of creating a shared context takes a quite different form in the classroom. An example of the school-grounded process can be seen in the initial lines of the current events dialogue presented earlier (Peshkin, 1978, p. 102):

Teacher: OK, current events. Glenn?
Student: Pablo Casals, the well-known cellist, died at ninety-six.
Teacher: OK, shush! Jim?
Student: The war over in the Middle East is still going on.
Teacher: Is it going on in the same way? Frank?

In the first utterance, the teacher attempts to establish the topic in a clear, though terse, manner. Its development, however, takes a rather peculiar form. The teacher's second utterance is markedly different from the third utterance, even though both utterances are responses to well-meaning and well-formulated statements on the part of the two students. Although it is not made explicit, it is evident that the teacher's response to Jim is one of acceptance while the response to Glenn is one of nonacceptance.

The differential acceptance, in turn, implies that there is more to the teacher's question than "meets the ear." The teacher asks for a discussion on current events, with no qualification added to the term. Nevertheless, the teacher's responses indicate that what is wanted is information concentrating on the latest international conflict, which is a highly qualified subset of current events. This is not stated, however, in the opening question or in the *have been some important new developments in relation to the crisis in the Middle East. I'd like to discuss this in our current events session today. Can anyone tell me what the latest reports have been?*)

2. When students' responses reflect misunderstanding of the issues at hand or of the teacher's intentions, then there should be an explicit and immediate clarification of the problem. (For example, to Glenn's response, the teacher might have said, *Your're right. That did happen, but when I was talking about current events, I really was thinking about some of the international relations issues. . . .*)

An interesting feature of these strategies is that they require the teacher to go beyond the question format and use extended comments. These comments serve to capture and reflect the social links that must exist in any chain of effective communication. Interestingly, in the teacher–child exchanges recorded in the literature, the absence of comments is striking (see Graesser & Black, 1985, for a recent compilation). The concentration on questions has been so excessive that it has led educators to minimize alternative modes of expression. Other modes are not only part of effective human communication, but they are often much *more suited* than questions to conveying the intentions and ideas that teachers wish to impart.

Using questions to avoid explicit criticism

One of the givens of the social context of the classroom is that the teacher and stu-

dents each have distinctly different roles. The teacher, as the expert, has both the right and the responsibility to *initiate* and thereby direct the educational exchange. By contrast, the students, as novices, primarily play the *responder* role, following the lead set by the teacher. The distinction between initiating and responding has powerful implications that are apparent throughout any dialogue.

A major consequence of the distinction is apparent with utterances containing "wrong information." Consider the situation where a young child, in the *initiating* role, explores the boundaries of a concept by asking a question such as *Do ducks have to wear boots in the rain?* The charm and inquisitiveness of the child's initiation makes it almost impossible for the adult to impart any response that contains even the hint of a negative affect. When the child's utterance is a *response* to a question initiated by an adult, however, the situation is entirely different. For example, a teacher may hold up a plate and ask *What is this?* Even to this simple question, a wide array of appropriate responses is possible (e.g., *a dish, something you eat with, a round thing*). However, no matter how great a teacher's range of acceptance, there is inevitably a set of responses that are inappropriate (e.g., "*I can make that into a hat*") and hence unacceptable. Thus "incorrect" utterances in the responder role are somehow not as acceptable as they may be in the initiator role.

The situation becomes particularly complex with young children. An important and positive result of the preschool movement was the recognition of the validity of the child's perspective. Teachers were encouraged to accept the wide array of "surprising" children's verbalizations, both in initiating and in responding roles. In practice, however, teachers face a dilemma. As human beings their "instinctive" reaction is to reject an incorrect response; on the other hand, they are told not to show their nonacceptance by telling the child he or she is wrong. The typical solution has been circuitous and basically unsatisfactory. The following examples illustrate some common coping mechanisms. (The excerpts are taken from a lesson in a Scottish classroom in which the teacher is asking 4-year-olds to group objects by whether they are rough or smooth.)

Example 1

Child: (picks up a rolling pin)
  Teacher: What's this, Brenda?
Brenda: (timidly) A bottle *(Note: In Brenda's home, milk bottles were used as rolling pins, a common practice in Scotland.)*
Teacher: A bottle? Is it? What is it?

Example 2

Teacher: *(after having established that the object was a rolling pin)* Where are you going to put the rolling pin, Joanne?
Joanne: (pointing to the "rough" ring) In there.
Teacher: Oh, Andrew. Is it all right if I put it in there?
Andrew: No.
Teacher: Where am I to put it?
Andrew: There *(pointing to the "smooth" ring)*.

Example 3

Teacher: *(referring to some soap the child has selected)* Do you wash you hands and your face in the morning?
Roger: (shakes head)

Teacher: You don't wash your face? What do you have to do with the soap?
Roger: Your hands.
Teacher: What else do you need to wash with?
Roger: A sponge.
Teacher: A sponge? *(turns to Linda)* What else would he need? What would he use to dry his face? Linda?
Linda: A towel.
Teacher: A towel. Roger, where will we put this soap? In beside the smooth ring or in the rough ring?
Roger: In the rough ring.
Teacher: In the rough ring? *(takes the soap from Roger)* Look, Brenda, you feel this. Is it smooth or is it rough?

As these examples illustrate, the teacher has difficulty observing the injunction of accepting "any" answer. At the same time, she studiously observes the injunction not to criticize overtly. Her escape from the dilemma is either to ask the question again using an incredulous tone or to ask another child in the hope of attaining a correct response. In both cases, explicit criticism has been avoided. However, the far more painful and confusing experience of implicit criticism is clearly present. Interestingly, this pattern is not confined to interchanges with preschool children. For example, a variant of this pattern is apparent in the jungle fire dialogue, in which the incoherent first response of an older student leads the teacher to ask incredulously, *You mean the grass gets on fire because the animals stay in the jungle?*

It goes without saying that this type of exchange is unpleasant and unrewarding for both adult and child. Ironically, the exchange is a direct consequence of interfacing nonsocial and social strategies. While the *nonsocial domain* requires the teacher to ask questions, the *social domain* requires the teacher to avoid explicit criticism. The effort to reconcile the two domains leads to situations that are more painful than those the injunctions were initially intended to avoid. As is so often the case, a situation that is unfortunate for any child is almost unbearable for learning-disabled children, given the insecurities and failures that they face elsewhere.

Fortunately, a solution exists that is not at all difficult although it may seem harsh. Specifically, when a child offers clearly wrong information, the teacher should state explicitly that the answer is incorrect. This method serves to bring the child back to the topic at hand. In the long run, explicit criticism is less painful and more constructive than questioning that carries implicit criticism. (For example, in the jungle fire dialogue, when the teacher asked, *How could grass in a jungle get on fire?* the child replied, *'Cause they have to stay in the jungle.* Rather than asking with an incredulous tone, a question that repeats the child's wrong response, the

teacher could have said, *They may have to stay in the jungle, but that has nothing to do with the fire getting started . . .*). She could then proceed with simplifying statements and questions to help the child approach the concept she wishes to teach.

•   •   •

The examples given here by no means exhaust the problems posed by the use or misuse of questions in the classroom. Likewise, the proposed solutions do not cover all the changes that are required if classroom dialogue is to be enhanced. They do serve, however, to illustrate the need to analyze and contain the role of questions in the school. Questions have become the staple of the classroom, but they cannot possibly take the burden of all the demands that are currently placed on them. By understanding what questions cannot accomplish, teachers can begin to use questions in more appropriate ways to achieve the goals that they can serve. Questions need not be abandoned; rather their misuses should be curbed so that constructive uses can emerge.

REFERENCES

Bellack, A.A., Kliebard, H.M., Hyman, R.T., & Smith, F.L. (1966). *The language of the classroom.* New York: Teachers College Press.

Blank, M. (1975). Verbalization from young children in experimental tasks. *Child Development, 46,* 254–257.

Blank, M., Rose, S.A., & Berlin, L. (1978a). *The language of learning: The preschool years.* New York: Grune & Stratton.

Blank, M., Rose, S.A., & Berlin, L. (1978b). *Preschool language assessment instrument.* New York: Grune & Stratton.

Bloom, B.S. (1976). *Human characteristics and school learning.* New York: McGraw-Hill.

Dillon, J.T. (1982a). The effect of questions in education and other enterprises. *Journal of Curriculum Studies, 14,* 127–152.

Dillon, J.T. (1982b). The multidisciplinary study of questioning. *Journal of Educational Psychology, 74,* 147–165.

Flanders, N. (1970). *Analyzing teaching behavior.* Reading, MA: Addison-Wesley.

Graesser, A.C., & Black, J.B. (Eds.). (1985). *The psychology of questions.* Hillsdale, NJ: Erlbaum.

Hoffman, M.L. (1981). Perspectives on the difference between understanding people and understanding things. In J.H. Flavell & L. Ross (Eds.), *Social cognitive development*. Cambridge, MA: Cambridge University Press.

Mishler, E.G. (1978). Studies in dialogue and discourse: III. Utterance structure and utterance function in interrogative sequences. *Journal of Reading Research, 7,* 279–505.

Parnell, M.M., Patterson, S.S., & Harding, M.A. (1984). Answers to Wh-questions: A developmental study. *Journal of Speech and Hearing Research, 27,* 297–305.

Peshkin, A. (1978). *Growing up American: Schooling and the survival of community*. Chicago: University of Chicago Press.

Pressley, M, & Forrest-Pressley, D. (1985). Questions and children's cognitive processing. In A.C. Graesser & J.B. Black (Eds.), *The psychology of questions*. Hillsdale, NJ: Erlbaum.

Shantz, C. (1975). The development of social cognition. In E.M. Hetherington (Ed.), *Review of child development research,* (Vol. 5). Chicago: University of Chicago Press.

Stevenson, H.W., Parker, T., Wilkinson, A., Bonnevaux, B., & Gonzalez, M. (1978). School, environment and cognitive development: A cross-cultural study. *Monographs of the Society for Research in Child Development, 43*(3), Serial No. 175.

Turiel, E. (1978). The development of concepts of social structure: Social convention. In J. Glick & K.A. Clarke-Stewart (Eds.), *The development of social understanding*. New York: Gardner Press.

Divergence and convergence between oral and written communication

Donald L. Rubin, PhD
Associate Professor
Department of Speech Communication
  and Department of Language
  Education
Fellow, Institute for Behavioral Research
The University of Georgia
Athens, Georgia

CURRENT INTEREST in the relation between speech and writing continues a venerable tradition. In *The Phaedrus*, Plato warned against the dangers of what was for his civilization a new-fangled technology. Writing, Plato feared, would erode the cultured Greek's well-developed capacity to commit information to memory. People would grow intellectually lazy relying on written records rather than on their own mental efforts. In addition, because writing gives life to a text apart from its author, Plato believed that writing would encourage insincere expression. Oral discourse, according to Plato, was not divorced in this way from the mind and heart of the speaker.

The cognitive psychologist Jerome Bruner (1966) was, like Plato, impressed by the profound differences between the processes of speaking and writing. But unlike Plato, Bruner regarded writing as the ultimate tool for thinking. To talk about an object or event requires the

Top Lang Disord, 1987, 7(4), 1–18
© 1987 Aspen Publishers, Inc.

speaker to abstract invariant, recurrent properties about that object or event. To write about an object or experience requires that the writer construct yet more abstract representations of a communication situation. The writer must also perform the task of abstractly representing the primary symbol system (oral) in terms of a secondary symbol system (written). Moreover, Bruner (1966), along with a host of contemporary educators and psychologists (e.g., Britton, Burgess, Martin, McLeod, & Rosen, 1975; Vygotsky, 1978), noted that the act of writing promotes thinking and learning in at least two ways:

1. By providing a permanent visual trace, writing allows the writer to review and reflect on the ideas already generated. In this sense, writing serves as an adjunct to short- and long-term memory.

2. Because it takes more time to write something than to say it, writing enhances opportunities for planning. This planning may encourage thinking of a particularly high order of creativity and organization. (But see Scardamalia and Bereiter, 1985, for the argument that the mere act of writing does not itself guarantee advanced cognitive processing.)

PERSPECTIVES ON ORAL AND WRITTEN LANGUAGE

Mounting evidence warrants acceptance of both Plato's and Bruner's claims about the relations between speech and writing. Cross-cultural studies corroborate Plato's notion that writing promotes a consciousness in which communicators are psychologically distanced from their subjects. Even preliterate children from writing-based cultures may be imbued with literate consciousness; thus, for example, they relate personal narratives in a third-person voice. Children from oral-based cultures consider it aberrant to transform first-person experience to third-person language (Scollon & Scollon, 1981).

Other cultural and historical studies lend credence to the cognitive psychologists' position that literacy is concomitant to a linear and analytical style of thought. Indeed, some scholars claim that Plato would hardly have been able to engage in ruminations of such an abstract nature had he not been born into a society that had refined and adopted an alphabetic writing system (Ong, 1982).

Plato and Bruner are also both correct in the fundamental position that they hold in common: Writing and speech are not merely alternative and equivalent ways of encoding language. Oral and written communication differ profoundly in both functional and structural properties.

An illustrative case: Divergent oral and written styles among speakers of nonstandard dialects

As an initial demonstration of the ways in which oral and written language diverge, consider the writing of speakers of nonstandard dialects. If people wrote as they spoke, one would expect to find clear evidence of dialect interference in writing. The bulk of empirical evidence contradicts this expectation.

Several studies compared the writing of Black English Vernacular (BEV) speakers with the writing of Standard English (SE) speakers; others compared oral and written productions of the same BEV speakers (see reviews of this literature in Hartwell [1980] and Piché, Rubin, Turner, & Michlin [1978]). The results of these sociolinguistic analyses overwhelmingly support several counterintuitive conclusions:

- The incidence of BEV features is much lower in writing than it is in speech.
- The kinds of BEV features that do slip into writing are usually morphological (e.g., deleted possessive markers, deleted third-person singular /-s/ on verbs), rather than more highly stigmatized syntactic features (e.g., multiple negation, pronominal apposition, such as "My brother he goes to . . .").
- The kinds of writing errors that BEV speakers produce differ little from the kinds of errors that otherwise comparable SE speakers are liable to commit.

In fact, no one is a native speaker of writing, not SE speakers and not BEV speakers. All novice writers must learn to switch into the written code, and nonstandard-dialect speakers are about as successful (or unsuccessful) as any others.

Although there may be few objective linguistic differences between the writing of nonstandard-dialect speakers and that of standard-dialect speakers, instructors may be more sensitive to the errors that appear in the writing of nonstandard-dialect speakers. They expect to find errors, and so they do. In one study, teachers were unable to differentiate with any accuracy papers typical of BEV writers from those typical of SE writers. However, when they attributed authorship of a paper to a BEV writer (whether or not that paper truly contained BEV features), they judged the writing quality more harshly than they did the same paper when they attributed it to an SE speaker (Piché et al., 1978).

Overview

What is true of the relation between oral and written language for speakers of nonstandard dialects is equally true for members of all speech communities: Writing is not merely speech set down in print. The following section of this article explicates in greater detail the manner in which spoken and written language diverge. Specific linguistic and textual features that characterize prototypical oral and written styles are presented. These stylistic features are seen as adaptations to characteristic features of oral and written communication contexts. One especially important distinction between oral and written contexts pertains to the nature of listening audiences as opposed to that of reading audiences.

Although spoken and written styles diverge in specifiable ways, for mature and expert communicators speech and writing converge in certain respects. This convergence is the subject of another section of this article. Among novice writers,

Although spoken and written styles diverge in specifiable ways, for mature and expert communicators speech and writing converge in certain respects.

written language is regarded as an alien and unnatural code bearing little resemblance to comfortable conversational language. This posture results in stilted, hypercorrect expression. More experienced writers, in contrast, temper their writing with orality as a way of establishing authorial voice and rapport with readers.

The final section of this article discusses some important ways in which talk can support learning to write. Structured oral communication experiences can accompany composing processes, can serve as adjuncts to composing, or can serve as cognitive calisthenics for developing skills that underlie writing ability, like audience adaptation.

DIVERGENCE BETWEEN ORAL AND WRITTEN CONTEXTS, ORAL AND WRITTEN STYLES

An individual who is literate sometimes writes and sometimes talks. D. Rubin (1984a) discussed channel of communication as one constituent of communicative contexts that affects a communicator's style across a wide range of stylistic features. In this sense, individuals are regarded as switching between oral and written codes much as bilingual speakers switch between distinct languages and bidialectal speakers switch between distinct dialects in response to the demands of communication situations. Learning to use oral and written language in situationally appropriate ways is part of the task of becoming communicatively competent within one's culture.

An example of code-switching between speech and writing

To visualize how the distinctive features of oral and written language appear in actual discourse, consider the following speech sample produced by a high school junior. In the sample, she is participating in a simulated job interview. The interviewer has asked her to tell about the extracurricular activities she has listed on her job application.

Okay. Ahm, this year is my first year in National Beta Club. In the regular Beta Club. I was involved in the Junior Beta Club several years ago. You know, whenever. Then in gymnastics I [sentence trail-off]. The season is generally from right after Christmas. Or we start practicing before Christmas usually. This year we got started late, but [sentence trail-off]. Ahm, it's my second year. And it lasts generally nearly to the end of school. Ahm, did I say this was my second year? [Interviewer: Uh hum.] This is my first year of competing. But ahm [sentence trail-off] I—like doing the bars. Par—uneven parallel bars. And the balance beam. And [sentence trail-off]. Spanish Club. This is my second year in Spanish Club. In order to be in it you have to take Spanish. And this is my second year of Spanish. And I guess that's about it.

In some respects, this passage represents a very unusual oral performance. It contains 128 words within two conversational turns (by standard counting rules). A typical conversational turn is about 10 words (Scardamalia, Bereiter, & Goelman, 1982). The text is responsive to the question posed, that is, coherent; but it is not very cohesive. Its fragmented organization, bursting forth in fits and starts, is in this respect quite characteristic of oral style.

Counting elliptical sentences (of which there are seven), the passage contains 20 T-units (minimal terminable units)(Hunt, 1970). Each T-unit except the final one consists of a single main clause. Sentences are loosely coordinated (there are nine coordinating conjunctions, including two adversative *buts* that the speaker was apparently unable to connect to any adversative propositional content) or merely juxtaposed, sometimes jarringly so.

The passage contains but a single subordinate clause, the noun clause "that's about it" functioning as a complement. Moreover, it appears more as a classic oral formula than as a complex grammatical structure. Note also the high frequency of hedges ("whenever," "generally," "usually"). The hedges, along with the speaker's false starts and self-corrections, contribute to the provisional tone of this response, although the student here is speaking of her own recent experiences.

This same girl produced the following writing sample in response to a portion of the job application form that asked her to describe what she considered an ideal job.

The perfect job for me would be a doctor with a few changes. I would enjoy the relationship between myself and my patients and I like the responsibility it would give me. My only changes would be that I need to work my hours into a schedule which would also allow me time for a family. I love children and enjoy working with them. A pediatrician would be most suited to me. I love to make people feel better and I'm willing to work for it. I don't mind schooling and I am quite adapted to it.

The reader's immediate impression of this writing sample is that it flows more smoothly and it is more integrated than the speech sample that precedes it. Lexical ties spanning clause boundaries contribute to this sense of cohesion (doctor ... patient; family ... child ... pediatrician). Endophoric pronoun references (i.e., references in which the referent is explicitly named in the text) also link sentences (relationship ... it; children ... them; to make people feel better ... it; schooling ... it). The prepositional phrase "with a few changes" that appears in the opening sentence, though perhaps graceless with respect to diction, presages the secondary theme of this piece of writing and therefore integrates it. It is also an example of integrated syntax, combining propositions in units smaller than a clause.

With its frequent coordinated clauses and its admittedly self-expressive tone (the latter a function of the assigned topic), this writing sample retains certain elements of an oral style. Note that this verbal, as opposed to heavily nominalized, style is a strength of this student's writing. Still, the sample contains longer T-units (10 main clauses in 99 words) and a greater density of subordination (3 subordinate clauses, including 2 within a single sentence) than the student's speech. Note, too, the attempt to establish subjunctive mood. Clearly this young writer differentiates between oral and written language.

Production parameters, communicative contexts, and stylistic features

In geometry and other branches of mathematics, proofs are constructed by building theorems from basic axioms and building corollaries from theorems. The relations among production, context, and style in speech and in writing are organized in an analogous manner.

The particular *stylistic features* that distinguish oral or written language (e.g., subordinating as opposed to coordinating conjunctions) are like corollaries that follow from—are contingent upon—certain aspects of oral or written communication contexts. For example, prototypical speech contexts (i.e., spontaneous face-to-face conversation between people who are intimately acquainted) are associated with self-expressive and social functions. In contrast, prototypical writing contexts (i.e., solitary writing for a largely unknown and anonymous readership) are associated with the goals of expressing logical or propositional content (Olson & Torrance, 1981). These *contextual factors* are like theorems, and they in turn derive from certain axioms. It is axiomatic that speech and writing differ in *production parameters*. For example, writers typically are able to produce their texts over a period of time, reflecting, drafting, and revising with a tempo that will not be directly represented in the final text that a reader reads. In contrast, face-to-face conversationalists work with an ephemeral medium and must compose their texts spontaneously in "real time."

Tables 1 and 2 illustrate the manner in which characteristics of oral and written styles are the consequences of prototypical oral and written communication contexts. The distinctive properties of these contexts, in turn, result from the constraints imposed by the ways in which people produce speech and writing.

Consider, by way of illustration, the often observed assertion that oral language can be context dependent, whereas written texts must be autonomous, or context independent (Hirsch, 1977; Olson, 1977). Because speaker and listener share a common physical and temporal context, speakers can appropriately refer to objects using deictic pronouns (e.g., "That's an abomination") and personal pronouns that have no antecedents in text, but that do have clear referents in the environment (e.g., "That's an abomination he's hung on the wall over there"). In addition, speakers and listeners often share networks of other common experiences and associations. Speakers can exploit such shared knowledge and successfully communicate using terms that would prove opaque to eavesdroppers outside the interaction (e.g., "Oh, yeah? I know one that's even abominabler").

In prototypical writing, the writer can safely make fewer assumptions about understandings in common with the reader. All information necessary to interpret the text must be packaged within the text itself. Even seemingly minor matters, such as using the definite article *the* before unique reference has been established within the text, can convey to readers that something is amiss. Readers may feel like they have tuned in to a program already in progress (e.g., "*The* work of art that evokes emotional reactions is by Bosch," as opposed to "*One* work of art that . . . ," or "*A* work of art that . . . ").

Just as oral and written styles are ultimately determined by parameters relating to their respective modes of production, so is each style consummately suited for its respective mode of reception (D. Rubin & Rafoth, 1986). That is, written language is (or ought to be) readable, and oral language is (or ought to be) listenable.

Listeners process the stream of speech

Table 1. Relations between production, context, and style in oral communication

Production parameters	Contextual factors	Stylistic features
Speaker and listener face-to-face	Tangible audience	First-person reference
	Immediate feedback	Second-person address
	Dynamic shifting between speaking and listening roles	Ellipses, sentence fragments
	Primarily expressive and social functions	Brief stretches of continuous discourse
	Speaker and listener share physical and temporal context	Exophoric reference (pronouns without textual antecedents)
	Parallel nonverbal channel	Semantic abbreviation (expressions invested with "insider" meaning)
Ephemeral message trace	Non–self-conscious, spontaneous	Gestural and paralinguistic modifiers and substitutions
Spontaneous, effortless production	Rapid rate of composition	High density of conjoined main clauses
	Rate of listener uptake corresponds to rate of speaker production	Lexical and thematic redundancy
		Vestigial interjections (e.g., "Oh," "well"), rhetorical interrogatives (e.g., "you know"), and other devices for maintaining the floor while thinking ahead
		Thematic digression
		Relatively short clauses with few nominalizations or participials
		Simple discourse structures, units resolved without embedding
		Conventions of oral diction (e.g., passive auxiliary "got," high frequency of Anglo-Saxon vocabulary, formulaic expressions, contractions, sentences with final prepositions)

much as speakers produce it. Neither has the luxury of recursive reflection, of returning to preceding portions of the text and reprocessing them before turning to a fresh portion of text. It is easier for speakers to produce strung-along, coordinated syntax. Likewise, it is easier for listeners to comprehend those sorts of constructions in which it is unnecessary to parse out embedded clauses or discontinuous dependencies.

Speech is redundant in part because repetition and paraphrase ease the speaker's burden of inventing subject matter on the run. Fortunately, redundancy is also well suited to the needs of listeners, who are generally unable to control the pace at which they must process the flow of infor-

Table 2. Relations between production, context, and style in written communication

Production parameters	Contextual factors	Stylistic features
Physical and temporal separation between writer and reader	Indeterminate audience diffuse in time and space	Topics and comments rendered explicit
	Writer anticipates reader responses in the face of delayed or no feedback	Extended monologue
		Cohesion established over long stretch of discourse
	Functions oriented toward conveying propositional content	Endophoric reference (pronoun antecedents within text)
	Graphic channel only	Explicit organizational cues to guide reader processing (transition statements, internal summaries, headings)
		Orthographic markers to disambiguate boundaries between idea units (punctuation, paragraphing)
Permanent message trace	Writer rescans text periodically, engages in recursive revision	High density of subordinate clauses
		Lexical diversity
		Thematic unity
Production requires planning, deliberate effort	Act of composing can extend over long time span, transcribing can be interrupted and resumed	Linear organization, little repetition
	Text is available to anonymous readers	Relatively long clauses integrate propositions by means of nominalization, participials
	Slow rate of composition	Authoritative tone (e.g., use of "indeed," "clearly")
	Writer attends to form	Relatively complex discourse structures, including embedded episodes, chained arguments
	Rate of reader uptake independent of rate of production	Word-order "inversions" (e.g., "To the ale house he strode")
		Conventions of written diction (e.g., high frequency of Latinate vocabulary, passive auxiliary "BE," subjunctive mood)

Speech is redundant in part because repetition and paraphrase ease the speaker's burden of inventing subject matter on the run.

mation, often distracted by environmental elements, and sometimes forced to cope with a degraded sound signal. Redundancy allows listeners to recover a once lost meaning the second time around. Indeed, orality in language is a primary factor contributing to listenability. Diagnostic, evaluative, or research instruments intended to specifically measure listening skills must use passages composed of oral language and not merely present written language through the auditory channel (Redeker, 1984: A. Rubin, 1980; D. Rubin & Rafoth, 1986).

Audience awareness

In everyday conversation each of us is liable to fall into occasional egocentric lapses and thus in one way or another fail to produce discourse that is adapted to our listeners. We may begin a conversation about some topic that has been preoccupying us without adequately setting the topical foundation for our listener (e.g., "You know what really bothers me about that painting?"; "But darling, you're the one who insisted we do the entire house in off-white"). Or we may attempt to persuade our listeners to follow some plan of action using arguments geared toward our own values rather than those of our targets.

However, in dialogue, we have the advantage of instantaneous feedback from our listeners, coupled with ongoing opportunities to modify our messages. We can, for example, append a definition (e.g., "No, no, when I said 'painting' I was talking about that Bosch piece hanging in the dentist's office") or an analogy (e.g., "I mean, you wouldn't hang a picture of Hercules and the Medusa in your bathroom, would you?").

Egocentric intrusions into conversations, therefore, are repairable; such intrusions into written monologue are not. Much as writers might wish that they could retract or alter what they have written, once cast out for audience consumption, written messages are immutable (but see Elbow, 1985, for an opposing point of view). As they compose, writers must constantly place themselves in the roles of readers who are naive to the writers' own intentions and meanings, readers who are likewise ignorant of the particular physical and temporal setting in which the writer composes (D. Rubin, 1984b).

Because the writer's audience is generally indeterminate ("the writer's audience is always a fiction" according to Ong, 1975), the task of representing one's audience to oneself is that much more difficult in writing as compared with speech (Kroll, 1978). For this reason, social cognition—the process of inferring others' thoughts, feelings, and beliefs—may be even more crucial to effective writing than it is to effective oral communication (Pellegrini, Galda, & Rubin, 1984b).

Social cognition, or more specifically, audience awareness, is central to writing persuasive arguments (choosing warrants, anticipating and refuting reservations), to knowing where and what kinds of elaboration to insert in a text (examples, paraphrases, references to authorities), and to producing intelligible syntax (endophoric pronoun reference, modifiers that do not dangle). Revision, in particular, requires that writers step outside their own egocentric perspectives on their texts and regard their writing with the fresh eyes of a reader naive to their intentions.

The lists of distinctive oral and written stylistic features presented in Tables 1 and 2, which are by no means exhaustive enumerations, are confirmed by analyses conducted by Horowitz and Newman (1964), O'Donnell (1974), A.Rubin (1980), Schafer (1981), Vachek (1973), and others. Recently, the work of Chafe (1982, 1985) has exerted considerable influence on research and theory regarding differences between oral and written communication (see Redeker, 1984; Tannen, 1985).

Chafe asserted that oral and written discourse differ across two dimensions: (1) involvement and (2) integration. The personal identification of speakers with their discourse is more apparent than the involvement of writers in theirs. The stylistic benchmark of prototypical essayistic writing—extended discursive exposition—is to disembody the written text from the writer. Thus, for example, passive constructions are more typical of writing than they are of speech (Chafe, 1985). At the same time, because the writer is freed of the tyranny of real-time composing, written texts can package information more compactly and in a more elaborately organized fashion than spoken texts can; they are more integrated. Writing, for example, generally manifests greater syntactic complexity than speech does (but

see Beaman, 1984, for some contrary evidence).

CONVERGENCE BETWEEN SPEAKING AND WRITING

To explicate the characteristic styles of speech and of writing, many analyses, like the speech/writing style presented earlier in this article, compare spontaneous conversational talk with more or less planned essay writing (Tannen, 1985). Even such comparisons between diametrically contrasting communication events reveal overlapping of the two styles. It is convenient to refer to a monolithic written style that is distinct from an equally monolithic oral style. Yet a more accurate portrayal refers instead to greater or lesser degrees of orality and literateness as dimensions that cut across all types of discourse, whatever the channel in which it is produced.

Composing speech in writing and writing in speech

Crystal and Davy (1969) pointed out that some works produced in writing are intended to be declaimed. Speech writers, in fact, are more likely to work with paper and pencil than with a tape recorder. By the same token, some speech is so utterly formulaic and intended "for the record" that it may as well be inscribed (e.g., the toasts offered back and forth between guests and hosts at diplomatic receptions).

Thus rather than being regarded as specific to one or the other channels of communication, oral and written styles can be thought of as opposing ends of a continuum. All discourse can be arrayed along the oral–written continuum (Tannen 1982; but see Tannen, 1985, for a revised formulation that holds "relative focus of interpersonal involvement" to be the definitive dimension), and the historical contingency of whether a particular piece of discourse arrives in print or in speech is not central to its essential orality or literate nature (D. Rubin & Rafoth, 1986).

Thus the language of written diary entries may resemble more the language of whispered intimacies between close friends than the language of academic essays. Similarly, the speech of an attorney arguing a brief before a court of appeals lies more at the written end of the continuum than does the writing of a gossip columnist in the daily newspaper.

Convergence, divergence, and reconvergence as the course of development in writing

Even very young children acquiring an initial sense of print do not treat the written code as an isomorphic reflection of oral communication (Harste, Woodward, & Burke, 1984). Yet in many respects the writing of inexperienced writers lies close to their speech.

Because of inexperienced writers' lack of familiarity with written language, because of the abstractness—and hence cognitive load—inherent in written communication contexts, and because of lapses in social cognition, features of oral language intrude with considerable detrimental effect in their writing. Thus, for example, the writing and speech of first graders show virtually indistinguishable frequencies of exophoric reference—

appropriate for speech but not for writing (King & Rentel, 1981; Pellegrini, Galda, & Rubin, 1984a). Shaughnessy (1977) and others found a similar convergence between the written and oral codes of adults who are inexperienced writers.

With more experience, writers learn to appropriately differentiate between speaking and writing (Kantor & Rubin, 1981). They build on linguistic and rhetorical skills acquired in speech, but they adapt them to meet the needs of readers (D. Rubin & Kantor, 1984). Conversational topic framers like "You know what's wrong with modern art these days?" provide the analogues to written topic framers like "Modern art in the final quarter of the 20th Century is plagued by three crises."

Experiences in adapting talk for listeners of varying backgrounds and statuses provide foundations for understanding how to write for a generalized, indeterminate readership. Strategies of oral persuasion like "Don't tell me that it's too much trouble to save your old newspapers, because I know you save lots of junk in your garage" are precursors to more elaborated strategies of written argumentation like "Opponents of the policy I am advocating have three major objections, but none of these can be shown to be valid."

This sort of differentiation between speech and writing is both normal and desirable. However, some inexperienced writers seem to pass through a stage in which they overcompensate for differences between speech and writing before they settle into the more normative patterns of differentiation. Such learners appear to operate according to an inner editor that tells them "I don't exactly know what written language is. But I do know that writing is different from speaking. So if it sounds anything like regular talk, it must be wrong. My job is to make this sound as little like comfortable speech as possible."

These writers may be said to hypercorrect when they switch from oral to written registers much as speakers of working–class dialects overshoot the upper–middle–class target when they attempt to switch to a formal speech register (Labov, 1972). Hypercorrect writing is produced by individuals who are well motivated in their intent to produce writing that is differentiated from speech, but who suffer from "linguistic insecurity" with respect to the written code. They are convinced that the style that feels right and that resembles their habitual writing must be wrong. Writers who hypercorrect aim for an unrealistic stereotype of what written language looks like, and the resulting prose is hackneyed, caricatured.

Hypercorrect writing includes many instances of malapropism (Wolfram & Whiteman, 1971). One high school writer, responding to the assignment to describe an ideal job, wrote, "I want a job that has alot of work. Like being a supervisor in constrution. I like a lot of hard work. I know I can work hard. I want a job that have alot of comprehension, and capability." Although "comprehension" and "capability" are indeed worthy aspirations, one must assume that what this student was really seeking in a job was "compensation" and "responsibility." He may have had a notion that somewhere in his essay he ought to use some multisyllabic words that somehow sound sophisticated, so he squeezed off a couple, and having done so, felt justified in regarding his work as complete.

Another type of lexical hypercorrection involves the use of expressions that inexperienced writers are likely to regard as literary formulas, but in fact are typically clichéd and vacuous. One example that is the bane of many examination graders is the seemingly irrepressible phrase, "In our modern world of today." Inexperienced writers are also likely to produce excess modifiers like "the actual truth of the matter" or coordinated complements like "This book is enjoyable and entertaining." Presumably, to novice writers these expressions "sound" like legalese (e.g., "necessary and sufficient," "does hereby obligate and bind"), which serves as an indisputable model for how written language is supposed to sound. In short, these writers are searching for that level of diction they believe functions as a conventional marker of literate style. However, because they remain aliens in the community of writers, their efforts result in hypercorrect forms that only confirm their lack of competence.

In addition to stereotyped expectations for the kinds of lexical choices that compose written language, many inexper-

Writers who hypercorrect aim for an unrealistic stereotype of what written language looks like, and the resulting prose is hackneyed, caricatured.

ienced writers have caricatured notions about the syntax of written language. Hypercorrect syntax is often marked by heavy nominalization and attempts at parallelism from which writers cannot disentangle themselves. Here is an example of hypercorrect syntax from a college junior's term paper:

The closeness of an extended family provides a consciousness of closeness to other without even having to verbally say anything, belongingness, and togetherness protects them. Communication within this extended family is equal with each member of the family having input into what is said and done with special attention given to a family member who might have special expertise concerning a particular problem or issue.

Competent writers do eventually learn how to properly differentiate between oral and written style. For those who develop further into expert, practiced writers, however, writing and speech reconverge (Kroll, 1981). For these writers, oral style becomes a resource that they judiciously draw on to evoke in readers a sense of interaction (D.Rubin & Rafoth, 1986). Aptly, literary analysts use words that refer to the world of orality to describe these stylistic impressions: *voice* and *tone*.

Consider this passage from Lewis Thomas's *The Lives of a Cell*, winner of a National Book Award for nonfiction:

I have been trying to think of the earth as a kind of organism, but it is no go. I cannot think of it this way. It is too big, too complex, with too many working parts lacking visible connections. The other night, driving through a hilly, wooded part of southern New England, I wondered about this. If not like an organism, what is it like, what is it *most* like? Then, satisfactorily for that moment, it came to me: it is *most* like a single cell. (Thomas, 1974, p. 4)

Here, Thomas "speaks" not with the authority of a writer, but with the provisionalism of a speaker. He creates the persona of an explorer groping his way from confusion to, if not Truth, at least satisfying explanation. The tone invites the reader to don a complementary role, the role of a colleague. Thomas achieves these effects most obviously by use of first person voice. (Elsewhere the book is written in the third person, but the tone remains colleagial.) Equally as effective, the passage includes conventionally oral diction ("no go"), digression ("driving through a hilly . . . "), redundancy ("what is it like, what is it *most* like?"), and even exophora to evoke a sense of immediacy ("the other night").

These devices for intruding orality into written texts are tools that accomplished writers use, not only to adapt to their audiences, but to create or define a relationship with their readers. They have constructed mental representations of their readers, of the role they want their readers to adopt. The stylistic features instantiate that role in the text.

Even in nonliterary genres like business correspondence and academic essays, accomplished writers exploit these resources to forge relationships of greater solidarity with their readers, to forge conversational relationships. They may use brief, uncluttered clauses. Or they may begin sentences with conjunctions to achieve a sense of dramatic pausing.

They'll intersperse an occasional contraction. Parenthetical expressions—like conversational asides uttered in a lower tone of voice—are set apart by punctuation or by lexical markers (e.g., "incidentally," "also germane to this point").

THE ROLE OF TALK IN WRITING INSTRUCTION

Knowledge about the nature of oral and written language points toward principled approaches for incorporating speech into writing instruction. The goal of such instruction would be to enable inexperienced writers to capitalize on the rhetorical prowess they have acquired in the more familiar oral channel. At the same time, they must learn to differentiate between oral and written language, to compare and contrast the two modes of communication.

Such instruction does not discount the value to students of becoming fluent and enthusiastic writers of orallike forms such as poetry, personal narrative, and casual correspondence. Indeed, students may be provided with deliberate practice in such forms, both because it will increase their pleasure and their competence in those particular genres and because those genres are transitional to other types of writing.

However, the ultimate test of whether such instruction succeeds is the students' mastery of less familiar forms of writing that diverge substantially from comfortable patterns of oral communication. These same forms, epitomized by the expository essay, also constitute (for better or for worse) the metric by which academic success is measured.

Skill domains

Table 3 (from D. Rubin & Dodd, in press) presents the variety of ways in which oral communication activities can support students' development toward the extended expository discourse that characterizes academic writing in most secondary and postsecondary schools. According to this analysis, inexperienced writers will need to extend their oral competencies to meet the demands of written communication in four domains.

First, writers need to *invent subject matter* in a monologic, internally cohesive fashion, without the scaffolding and presumption of shared understandings inherent in dialogue.

Second, broadly competent writers need to be able to *address remote and indeterminate audiences*. Unlike a conversational partner, the writer's audience works without the benefit of environmental and paralinguistic cues. Furthermore, listeners are generally obliged by prior interpersonal bonds with the speaker to invest energy in deciphering the message. A psychologically distant reader has little such motivation, and so the onus for intelligibility falls heavily on the writer (Shaughnessy, 1977).

Third, even the solitary writer who *engages in cooperative discourse*, participates in a broadly conceived conversation (Bazerman, 1980). Writers must tailor their writing to contribute to an ongoing accretion of knowledge about a topic. At the same time, they must conform to certain conventions that a community of writers and readers in a given genre have come to expect. For example, in a traditional high school or college term paper,

Table 3. Oral-based activities in composition instruction

Skill domain	Accompanying composing processes	Adjuncts to composing	Cognitive calisthenics
Invention—discovering subject matter, elaborating, forging topical coherence	Prewriting discussion, interviewing as an information gathering tool	Tape-recording notes, dictating "zero drafts"	Topic sculpting impromptus, forum questioning
Audience awareness—anticipating and adapting to the responses of readers with diverse backgrounds and to their informational and language processing needs	Helping circles, oral "publication," teacher conferencing	"Talk–write" dyads, audience interviews	Role-switching, discussing moral dilemmas
Cooperative discourse—building on what has been said before, both interacting with a particular audience and within a broader cultural context; being relevant, making a contribution, acknowledging sources	Group work in dividing a topic, group reports	Collaborative drafting, group revising	Instruction in listening, peer questioning as a tool for learning how to internalize dialogue
Monitoring—metacognitive awareness, reflecting on and distancing oneself from one's own discourse, adopting a critical stance	Reading aloud to facilitate editing, group critiques	Thinking-aloud composing, discourse-based interviews for self-assessment	Structured forensic discussion, transcribing speech

writers must document their information with citations to previous work. They are obliged to acknowledge areas of incompleteness in their reasoning both to invite public scrutiny and criticism and to offer promising directions to other members of the reading or writing community who might wish to carry the inquiry forward in the future.

Fourth, writers constantly *monitor their messages*, engage in ongoing and recursive revision, in a way that is not possible in speech. Although this monitoring inhibits fluency, it enables more precise expression. It also encourages writing's orientation toward propositional content rather than expressive involvement. Monitoring encourages objectification of thought, which is the distinctive mark of writing as a mode of thinking. Inexperienced writers may learn to engage in superficial monitoring, to detect errors in writing mechanics and the like, but their oral communication habits give them little experience in distancing themselves from their discourse in the way that academic writing demands.

Functions of oral activities

In addition to presenting four skill domains involved in transferring oral competence to written competence, Table 3 suggests that oral communication activities can help bridge the gap between oral and written competencies by performing any of three functions in writing instruction.

First, talk can *accompany* composing processes. Perhaps the most prevalent use of talk in writing classes is large-group prewriting discussion. The purpose of such discussions is to help students discover what they have to say about a topic, to aid in invention. The art of managing such discussions lies in knowing when to cut them off. If students have completely spent their ideas in talk, if they no longer feel any dissonance or uncertainty about an assigned topic, then they will not be motivated to write. A practice that can be used to avoid this danger, at least in part, calls for students to write, then to talk about ideas emerging but perhaps still inchoate in their compositions, then to resume writing.

Second, oral communication activities can also serve as an *adjunct* to composing. In such activities a portion of the composing process—planning or drafting or revising—is actually performed in speech. A well-known example of such a method is Zoellner's (1969) talk–write technique. In this procedure, students work in pairs, and the dialogue between writer and audience becomes transformed into a draft that the writer composes as the reader looks on. Dictation is a related technique. Very minimal cues that simulate a dialogic context (e.g., "Go on" or "Can you add anything to that?") can significantly increase inexperienced writers' output in dictation (Scardamalia, et al., 1982).

Third, oral activities can serve as *calisthenics* to promote cognitive abilities that underlie extended expository writing. The goal of these calistenics is not to serve as writing stimuli, though writing assignments can often be profitably posed at their conclusion. Rather, through repeated exposure to these structured exercises, students will build up their cognitive capacities in areas critical to higher-order literacy.

Role-switching activities (D. Rubin & Dodd, in press) require students to repeatedly engage in dramatic improvisations surrounding a single scenario (e.g., a scenario in which a college student seeking summer employment as a farm laborer encounters a migrant worker, a supervisor, and a consumer). Students take turns playing all the roles in the scenario so that they can experience each perspective. Role switching is intended to improve inexperienced writers' ability to appreciate divergent perspectives on a single

Role switching is intended to improve inexperienced writers' ability to appreciate divergent perspectives on a single event and thus increase their audience awareness.

event and thus increase their audience awareness.

• • •

Inexperienced writers grapple with the task of figuring out how writing works. In doing so, they are both helped and hindered by their reliance on oral communication—their primary mode of expression. If they are successful in their task, they will come to understand that oral and written language diverge in some respects and converge in others. However, it is not likely that they will attain this insight if instruction in writing is divorced from instruction in speech. Instructors can help inexperienced writers succeed by providing opportunities in which speech and writing can be directly compared, laying bare their conflicting demands, but also illuminating their mutual goal: communication.

REFERENCES

Bazerman, C. (1980). A relationship between reading and writing: The conversational model. *College English, 41,* 656–661.

Beaman, K. (1984). Coordination and subordination revisited: Syntactic complexity in spoken and written narrative discourse. In D. Tannen (Ed.), *Coherence in spoken and written discourse* (pp. 45–80). Norwood, NJ: Ablex.

Britton, J., Burgess, T., Martin, N., McLeod, A., & Rosen, H. (1975). *The development of writing abilities (11–18).* London: Macmillan Education.

Bruner, J.S. (1966). *Toward a theory of instruction.* Cambridge, MA: Harvard University Press.

Chafe, W. (1982). Integration and involvement in speaking, writing, and oral literature. In D. Tannen (Ed.), *Spoken and written language* (pp. 35–54). Norwood, NJ: Ablex.

Chafe, W. (1985). Linguistic differences produced by differences between speaking and writing. In D. Olson, N. Torrance, & A. Hildyard (Eds.), *Literacy, language, and learning* (pp. 105–124). Cambridge, England: Cambridge University Press.

Crystal, D., & Davy, D. (1969). *Investigating English style.* Bloomington, IN: Indiana University Press.

Elbow, P. (1985). The shifting relationships between speaking and writing. *College Composition and Communication, 36,* 283–304.

Harste, J.C., Woodward, V.A., & Burke, C.L. (1984). *Language stories and literacy lessons.* Portsmouth, NH: Heinemann.

Hartwell, P. (1980). Dialect interference in writing: A critical view. *Research in the Teaching of English, 14,* 101–118.

Hirsch, E.D. (1977). *The philosophy of composition.* Chicago: University of Chicago Press.

Horowitz, M.W., & Newman, J.B. (1964). Spoken and written expression: An experimental analysis. *Journal of Abnormal and Social Psychology, 68,* 640–647.

Hunt, K.W. (1970). Syntactic maturity in school children and adults. *Monographs of the Society for Research in Child Development, 35* (1, Serial No. 134).

Kantor, K.J., & Rubin, D.L. (1981). Between speaking and writing: Processes of differentiation. In B. Kroll & R. Vann (Eds.), *Exploring speaking–writing relationships: Connections and contrasts* (pp. 55–81). Urbana, IL: National Council of Teachers of English.

King, M., & Rentel, V. (1981). Research update: Conveying meaning in written texts. *Language Arts, 58,* 721–728.

Kroll, B.M. (1978). Cognitive egocentrism and the problem of audience awareness in written discourse. *Research in the Teaching of English, 12,* 269–281.

Kroll, B.M. (1981). Developmental relationships between speaking and writing. In B. Kroll & R. Vann (Eds.), *Exploring speaking–writing relationships: Connections and contrasts* (pp. 32–54). Urbana, IL: National Council of Teachers of English.

Labov, W. (1972). *Sociolinguistic patterns.* Philadelphia: University of Pennsylvania Press.

O'Donnell, R.C. (1974). Syntactic differences between speech and writing. *American Speech, 49*(1), 102–110.

Olson, D. (1977). From utterance to text: The bias of language in speech and writing. *Harvard Educational Review, 47,* 257–281.

Olson, D., & Torrance, N. (1981). Learning to meet the requirements of written text: Language development in the school years. In C. Frederikson & J. Dominic (Eds.), *Writing: The nature, development, and teaching of written communication* (pp. 235–255). Hillsdale, NJ: Erlbaum.

Ong, W. (1975). The writer's audience is always a fiction. *Publication of the Modern Language Association*, *90*(1), 9–21.

Ong, W. (1982). *Orality and literacy: The technologizing of the word*. New York: Methuen.

Pellegrini, A.D., Galda, L., & Rubin, D.L. (1984a).Context in text: The development of oral and written language in two genres. *Child Development*, *55*, 1549–1555.

Pellegrini, A.D., Galda, L., & Rubin, D.L. (1984b). Persuasion as a social cognitive activity: The effects of age and channel of communication on children's production of persuasive messages. *Language and Communication*, *4*, 285–293.

Piché, G.L., Rubin, D.L., Turner, L.J., & Michlin, M.L. (1978). Effects of nonstandard dialect features in written compositions on teachers' subjective evaluations of students and composition quality. *Research in the Teaching of English*, *12*, 107–118.

Redeker, G. (1984). On differences between spoken and written language. *Discourse Processes*, *7*(1), 43–55.

Rubin, A. (1980).A theoretical taxonomy of the differences between oral and written language. In R. Spiro, B. Bruce, & W. Brewer (Eds.), *Theoretical issues in reading comprehension* (pp. 411–438). Hillsdale, NJ: Erlbaum.

Rubin, D.L. (1984a). The influence of communicative context on style in writing. In A.D. Pellegrini & T. Yawkey (Eds.), *The development of oral and written language in social contexts* (pp. 213–232). Norwood, NJ: Ablex.

Rubin, D.L. (1984b). Social cognition and written communication. *Written Communication*, *1*, 211–245.

Rubin, D.L., & Dodd, W.M. (in press). *Talking into writing: Speech exercises for college basic writers*. Urbana, IL: ERIC Reading and Communications Skills Module and National Council of Teachers of English.

Rubin, D.L., & Kantor, K.J. (1984). Talking and writing: Building communication competence. In C. Thaiss & C. Suhor (Eds.), *Speaking and writing* (pp. 29–74). Urbana, IL: National Council of Teachers of English.

Rubin, D.L., & Rafoth, B.A. (1986). Oral language criteria for selecting listenable materials: An update for reading teachers and specialists. *Reading Psychology*, *7*, 137–152.

Schafer, J.C. (1981). The linguistic analysis of spoken and written texts. In B. Kroll & R. Vann (Eds.), *Exploring speaking–writing relationships: Connections and contrasts* (pp. 1–31). Urbana, IL: National Council of Teachers of English.

Scardamalia, M., & Bereiter, C. (1985). The development of dialogic processes in writing. In D. Olson, N. Torrance, & A. Hildyard (Eds.), *Literacy, language, and learning* (pp. 307–333). Cambridge, England: Cambridge University Press.

Scardamalia, M., Bereiter, C., & Goelman, H. (1982). The role of production factors in writing ability. In M. Nystrand (Ed.), *What writers know* (pp. 173–209). New York: Academic Press.

Scollon, R., & Scollon, J. (1981). *Narrative, literacy and face in interethnic communication*. Norwood, NJ: Ablex.

Shaughnessy, M. (1977). *Errors and expectations*. New York: Oxford University Press

Tannen, D. (1982). The oral/literate continuum of discourse. In D. Tannen (Ed.), *Spoken and written language* (pp. 1–16). Norwood, NJ: Ablex.

Tannen, D. (1985). Relative focus of involvement in oral and written discourse. In D. Olson, N. Torrance, & A. Hildyard (Eds.), *Literacy, language, and learning* (pp. 124–148). Cambridge, MA: Cambridge University Press.

Thomas, L. (1974). *The lives of a cell: Notes of a biology watcher*. New York: Bantam Books.

Vachek, J. (1973). *Written language: General problems and problems of English*. The Hague, Netherlands: Mouton.

Vygotsky, L. (1978). *Mind in society: the development of higher psychological processes*. Cambridge, MA: Harvard University Press.

Wolfram, W., & Whiteman, M. (1971). The role of dialect interference in composition. *Florida FL Reporter*, *9*(1,2), 34–38, 59.

Zoellner, R. (1969). Talk–write: A behavioral pedagogy for composition. *College English*, *30*, 267–320.

Part II
Language Assessment and Literacy Development

Ethnography and literacy: Learning in context

Andrea R. Fishman, PhD
Assistant Professor
Department of English
Associate Director
Pennsylvania Writing Project
West Chester University
West Chester, Pennsylvania

MUCH HAS BEEN learned from ethnographic research about literacy in the past twenty years. Through ethnography, lessons have been taught on the basis of social realities (Heath, 1983; Taylor & Dorsey-Gaines, 1988) as well as cognitive realities (Cole, 1981; Wagner, 1983). In ethnography, lessons have been learned from individuals (Bissex, 1980; Calkins, 1983), from classrooms (Mehan, 1979; Michaels, 1983; Perl & Wilson, 1986), and from communities (Cazden & John, 1971; Fishman, 1988; Heath, 1983). Always, however, the lessons in ethnography have been learned and taught in terms of their cultural contexts, whether those cultures are the commonly recognized sort—the inner city (Taylor & Dorsey-Gaines, 1988) or the Amish settlement (Fishman, 1988)—or the less commonly recognized variety—the home (Bissex, 1980) or the first grade classroom

Top Lang Disord, 1992,12(3),67–75
© 1992 Aspen Publishers, Inc.

(Michaels, 1983). In fact, the contention in ethnography is that meaning only exists in context; there is no other kind (Mischler, 1979).

To understand what a particular school, curriculum, teacher, or clinician intends to convey by the term *literacy*, therefore, can be neither assumed nor generalized. There are no typical schools, classrooms, teachers, or students from an ethnographic perspective. An understanding of literacy can only be attained through participant observation in the particular setting in question. Ethnographers strive to understand how other people see and understand the world, assuming, as Smith states, that "people always act rationally to make sense of the world they are experiencing [and that] repeated patterns of behavior are doing something positive" (D. Smith, Personal Communication, September 1982) for those who use them. In terms of literacy this means that people read and write in ways that are useful and make sense to them, regardless of how their reading and writing may appear to outsiders.

Achieving this sort of contextual understanding is, obviously, labor intensive. It requires time, effort, involvement, and energy far beyond that of traditional literacy-assessment instruments. So the question becomes, What makes ethnographic understanding worthwhile? Why should context be accounted for in assessing, analyzing, or describing a child's literacy?

The answer is that context counts because children do not learn to read and write in a vacuum; they do not even learn to read and write in a laboratory or other sorts of testing contexts. Rather, children learn to read and write in school and classroom settings where they learn the setting along with the skills. When children read and write, the literacy, or the lack of literacy, displayed may reflect four dimensions of their learning that are crucial to understanding their work:

1. Children's reading and writing may reflect what they have been taught to do more than what they are able to do.
2. Children's reading and writing may reflect what they know about more than what they are able to learn.
3. Students' literacy may reflect what they care or do not care about doing more than what they are able to do.
4. Children's literacy may reflect who they know and know how to relate to rather than who they could know and learn how to relate to.

Thus, if educators and clinicians are to have some impact on children's future literacy development through their intervention, they must understand why children read and write as they do and how those factors can be addressed and perhaps adjusted to facilitate further growth. In other words, children may have all the ability they need; the key to further literacy development may rest in the needs the context establishes for such children.

To illustrate the power of ethnography to contextualize and thereby expand the understanding of literacy, this article presents two case studies. Both of these eighth-grade students attend school in southeastern Pennsylvania. A portfolio of each student's work will display their literacy, followed by ethnographic contextualization, which will interpret that work in light of the particular setting in which it was produced.

CASE STUDY #1: DANIEL

Case study #1 is Daniel, and sample #1 examines his reading comprehension. Daniel read a story called, "The Joker." It is about a boy named Dennis Conron who, along with his friends, played practical jokes on a schoolmate until one "joke" backfired and they all learned a predictable lesson. The questions (Q) are from the test; the answers (A) are written by Daniel.

Q: What was the joke that the boys played on Eddie Davis?
A: moved the furniture into Charlies room
Q: Why did they choose Eddie to play it on? What does the word GULLIBLE mean?
A: they could make him believe things that aren't so, easily tricked
Q: What type of person was Dennis Conron? Use parts of the story as evidence for what you say.
A: short and cheerful,
Q: Do you feel Dennis could be blamed for Eddie's accident? Write a paragraph explaining your feelings on this.
A: yes,
Q: Did Eddie ever understand the joke? Explain.
A: yes, because the joker did it

What questions does this test raise about Daniel's literacy and his ability to understand what he reads, to write in complete sentences, to explain himself fully, and to follow directions? Perhaps more important than the questions this test raises, what are the answers it suggests to those questions? On the basis of this test, where would Daniel be placed? What language-arts objectives would be written for him? What kinds of reading and writing exercises would he be assigned? Results of an ethnographic analysis would neither draw attention to these questions, nor provide their answers. Rather, in an ethnographic analysis, first other reading and writing samples of Daniel's would be examined.

Sample #2 is a page from a social studies report Daniel wrote about Japan, the topic country assigned to him by his teacher. Daniel wrote 17 lined, loose-leaf pages, almost all with traced illustrations, a few with no text other than labels. The first page of "Japan" offered a map of the country marked with six major cities. The second page, headed "Weather," had one line of text—"Here is the weather in Japan."—and was divided in quarters, each containing an outline map color coded to illustrate "Average precipitation in August," "Average Yearly Precipitation," "Average temperatures in August," and "Average Precipitation in Feb."

The more extended written text appeared on pages separated by topic and labeled with headings "People," "Lands," "Work," "Education," "Minerals and Energy," and so forth. The page called "Education" read as follows:

Nearly all of Japans school-age children attend school regularly. Attendance is compulsory through the lower level of secondary school. Children begin nursery school when they are about 3. At 6, they begin elementary school; at 12, lower-secondary school.

Any student who has completed lower-secondary school may enroll in an upper-secondary school. The Japanese upper-secondary school is comparable to the United States high school. It offers either a technical or a college preparatory course of instruction.

Japanese students, especially those who plan to attend college, strongly compete with each other for grades and honors.

Sample #3 is a composition Daniel wrote about his pet in response to his teacher's directive to write three paragraphs describing the animal, giving its good and bad habits, and "telling what its future is." Daniel wrote about his horse, Rex.

Rex
He is brown and black mixed. He is about six feet tall. I have him around half a year.

His good habits are he doesn't kick and his bad habits are he tries to bite you. He doesn't follow me arround. I din't have him long enough to see how he got along with other horses.

The future of him is Rex and I are going to live together in an old shack.

Sample #4 is a letter Daniel wrote to me when I was a participant-observer in his school and asked all the students to write, telling me what they thought I ought to know. Daniel wrote:

Dear Andy,

We play kickball at recess. The name of the ball is "Big Kick" it is very light. Today, March 31, 1983, we played Amish against the Mennonite. I don't know who won yet because we didn't have last recess yet.

We give a newspaper out every first of the month. The name of the newspaper is "Meadow Brook Gazette." We each had to give a title to Verna Z. Burkholder. She looked over each one to see which one was the best. A sixth grader won, Marlin Martin. And whoever had something to do with Meadow Brook got a prize.

There are two first graders, five second graders, one third grader, three fourth graders, five fifth graders, two sixth graders, two seventh graders, and three eighth graders. They average up to about twenty with the teacher. We have about four weeks of school left. And I'm the happiest boy alive!

By looking at these samples of Daniel's work, can Daniel's literacy now be described, analyzed, and assessed? More information about his reading and writing can be obtained from all these samples than from a single test, and the range of skills and strategies evident in these samples is considerable, from the three-word answer to the opening reading comprehension question to the apparent plagiarism of the Japan report to the voiceless composition about Rex to the not-so-voiceless letter to me. So what conclusions can be drawn about Daniel and his literacy from all these samples? None yet, ethnographers would reply. Although a portfolio of Daniel's work has been examined, the context—the culture—that called forth these pieces has not been considered.

Daniel is Daniel Fisher, and he is the oldest of five children in an Old Order Amish family. His school, Meadow Brook, is operated by Pennsylvania's Old Order Amish community for the purpose of educating only Old Order Amish and Old Order Mennonite children. Daniel was one of three children in the eighth grade that year; they were the three oldest of 27 children enrolled in this first-through-eighth-grade one-room school.

As an ethnographer, I was a participant-observer in Meadow Brook school almost daily for six months. A few of the many things I learned about the Amish through these experiences include the following:

1. All texts are read as true, beginning with the Bible and extending to all others. The Amish have no concept of fiction, even though what is known in American literature as fiction is read.

2. The dominant mode of instruction is modeling—teacher for students, older students for younger ones. Children do what they see others doing.

3. Accuracy matters; appearance does not.

4. Time is valuable and not to be wasted.

5. The group is more important than any individual, whether self or other.

What do these five observations have to do with understanding Daniel's literacy? A great deal. Daniel, like his classmates, answers questions as asked and does work as assigned. He states facts as accurately and as briefly as possible, not wasting time explaining, supporting, or rewording information that is perfectly clear as stated. His reading textbook may want "evidence," but he knows his culture does not require any. Plagiarism also is not a problem with which his culture is concerned. Plagiarism is not an Amish concept. No Amish writers would ever attempt to claim another's words as their own, for they have no reason to. Neither fresh style nor original ideas are valued by this culture; getting work done as effectively, efficiently, and accurately as possible is. No Amish want to stand out from the group; they want only to be a part of it.

So is Daniel lazy, unoriginal, less than bright, or dishonest? Not at all. Is he literate according to the definition of his school? Most definitely. He is even sophisticated enough to adjust his literacy to his audience as he did in his letter to me. Does he work hard? Absolutely. He does all his work in precisely the fashion demanded. Does he need remediation, tutoring, or a resource room to bring him up to grade level or help him cope? No. Daniel was looked up to and emulated by all the younger boys at Meadow Brook because he was such a good Amishman.

CASE STUDY #2: MITCH

To test his reading comprehension, Mitch also was asked to answer questions about a story he had read. Mitch's story was called "On The Run." It was about Duke, a boy who was sent to a court-operated residential facility, Highland Hills, for stealing a car. Again, the questions (Q) are from the test; the answers (A) are the student's.

> Q: How does Duke feel about himself at the beginning? What clues tell you this?

> A: Duke feelt not sure about himself. He try to blam pass times on his actions.

> Q: How do Duke's feelings about himself influence the decisions he makes?

> A: He was blamming his pass on his crime the he did.

> Q: What is the idea behind a place like Highland Hills?

> A: To help you find yourself.

> Q: Why is it important to know who you are? What should you do with this knowledge?

> A: So you can take full responsablity for your actions.

> Q: If you met Duke, how would you feel about him?

> A: I will feel like he is learning his leson and is brave.

The curriculum at Mitch's school does not include report writing, so sample #2 of Mitch's literacy cannot parallel Daniel's. Instead, sample #2 for Mitch consists of his responses to arguments put forth by the reading comprehension testmaker with which he was to agree or disagree. Mitch was presented with three "arguments in favor of teenagers" and three "arguments in favor of adult authorities."

When presented with the statement, "Teenagers who have been in trouble understand each other's problems," Mitch was given three lines on which to respond. He wrote, "Yes becous thay been throw the same thing. Plus they know what's going on at the time," taking up all three lines. When presented with the statement, "People need to be educated to understand teenage problems" and given three more lines on which to respond, Mitch filled all three, writing, "Yes, thay wear teenage befor, but this time is changing faster than ever."

Sample #3 comes from the reading

workshop in which Mitch participates each Friday in English class. There students choose their own texts from a classroom library of books, magazines, and newspapers, and they write about what they have read in black-and-white composition books they call their reading logs.

The teacher's instructions for keeping the log say,

> Tell me what you have read. . . . you must write something even if it is only a couple of words. Try to tell me what you thought about what you read and why. Tell me if you liked or didn't like it and why. Tell me if it meant anything to you or if it stunk and why . . . share your experiences, ideas or questions.

The log entries are often addressed to the teacher directly.

In reading workshop, Mitch can pursue his own interests, raise his own issues, and has unlimited space in his log and fewer constraints on what he may say.

One day Mitch wrote:

> I just read a short articol from Yo magazin. It was about my budy Ice Cube [a currently popular rap musician]. He was tell Yo about the death threats. He say rapper live day by day with them. But he not sceared. In fact he named his new LP Kill at Will. I think the people that give these threat are just shoud jump off a brig, becose they are just jeleas.

Sample #4 for Mitch is also a letter. Through his English teacher, Mitch became pen pals with a student at an all-girls private Catholic school, Our Lady Academy. The Our Lady girls initiated the exchange, and Mitch received a letter from Andrea, who began their correspondence writing about her favorite and least favorite sports. Andrea then asked Mitch about his taste in sports and music. Mitch wrote back:

> Dear Andrea
>   My name is Mitchell thay call me the godfather. Im 17 years old but I still look a little younger than that. I like sports to, the sport I like is football. Im one of the best player in Brighton school. But the only sports that Brighton have is basketball, baseball, sofball, and track.
>   My favorite music is rap and hip hop on the R&B tip. My favorite rappers are Big Daddy Kane, Eric B and Hakim, LL Cool J, Ice Cube, N.W.A., EPMD, Public Enemy, 3rd Base, Special Ed and MC Lite. That should tell you something about me. ((I'm live as shit))
>   Im very wild out in the world but when Im in school I play the game. I do what thay want me to do when thay want me to do it. Im a very good student thay think. But when Im out Im another person. I make that change so I can be someone in life. I hope you understan this letter so far becous it hard putting things in words.
>   It aright up here its just like collage. Yes you have to do a crime to get up here. I hop nobody told you otherwise. Becous it would'nt be fair to you if you had the wrong idea that this is a regular school. We only go home every other weekend.
> P.S Wright back and send me a picher of you.
>   Im 5000 Jee
>   Stay safe
>   Godfather

By reading these samples of Mitch's work, some idea of the context in which he reads and writes can be appreciated, but, ethnographically, that is not quite enough. Instead of assessing, analyzing, or describing Mitch's literacy on this basis, an ethnographic analysis would focus more directly on the context of Mitch's learning, which is Brighton School.

Brighton is a residential school for adjudged and adjudicated juveniles, a school one hour and light-years away from Meadow Brook. Mitch is African American and from Philadelphia. He was sent to Brighton for breaking his probation on an assault charge for stealing cars. He had drugs in his possession when he was arrested, but his judge did not know he was also selling crack cocaine. Mitch's race, hometown, and drug and theft connections are shared by more than 95% of his schoolmates.

The differences between Brighton's culture and Meadow Brook's culture are as fascinating as the similarities between Brighton's literacy and Meadow Brook's literacy. Once again, these differences and similarities are accessible only through ethnography. Whereas Meadow Brook students do their work because their culture values inclusion, cooperation, and shared responsibility, Brighton students do their work because they will "lose points" if they do not, and enough points lost means no "home pass" on the next home pass weekend. The Brighton culture, in other words, values material reward and fears material punishment, neither of which are operative features of Meadow Brook School.

Similarly, whereas Meadow Brook students work diligently to avoid being singled out—to be as much like their peers as possible—Brighton students work so they can stand out from the rest. They love to compete—and to win—not as a team but as individuals. Much, if not most, of the work in Mitch's English class is cast as contests—to guess endings, to write the best ending, to read the most books—with winners receiving gum, M&M's, candy bars, or cola.

The environments of the two schools are notably different as well. Though both are rural, Meadow Brook is a stable, consistent, predictable environment in which people are quiet, respectful, and orderly at all times. Not only is there only one day off in the entire school calendar, but everyone is present and prompt nearly every day. School is work for these students, and

work is of value, worthy of everyone's best efforts.

Brighton, on the other hand, is constantly in flux. Not only are there students new to the school and to Mitch's English class nearly every week, but class members are often absent—called to see their social workers or judges, having run away or not returned from home pass or having been discharged or "shipped" (i.e., sent to more secure facilities). Unpredictability and instability are the rule at Brighton, not the exception. No matter who is present or absent, teasing, punching, threatening, and "going off" are daily occurrences in the classroom and in the halls. These students may be there together and may share an "us–them" mentality in relation to their teachers and society in general, but on a day-to-day, hour-to-hour basis, it is every individual for himself or herself.

Just as these contextual differences are marked and affect the ways literacy is used and defined, however, the same may be said of the similarities. The students at both Meadow Brook and Brighton do as much as necessary to meet assignment requirements and as little as they can to achieve the same ends. When asked through the use of textbook questions to use textual evidence to support their answers, whether that evidence is called "parts of the story" (Meadow Brook) or "clues" (Brighton), none feel compelled to comply. In other words, all these students "read" their assignments, their teachers, and their cultures perfectly. They know what is actually required, and they know what really is not necessary or valued. In the case samples cited, none of the writers lost credit for omitting specific evidence as requested by the text. None were penalized for omitting information, and none were penalized for the mechanical or grammatical errors in their work. Neither teacher corrected mistakes that did not interfere with meaning. Daniel's teacher, Verna Burkholder, represents a culture that values efficiency more than perfection; Mitch's teacher, Eileen Larkin, represents a culture that values communication and participation most. Verna avoids wasting time on perceived frills; Eileen avoids being perceived as caring more about punctuation errors than about people's honest efforts.

For Mitch, Daniel, and their classmates, self-selected reading is somehow different from the assigned variety. Just as the Meadow Brook students eagerly read and swap books during their spare time in school, Brighton students look forward to Fridays and object loudly if for some reason reading workshop is skipped. Just as reading for their own reasons is more enthusiastically pursued than other varieties, writing for their own reasons calls for more personal investment as well. Daniel could be more himself writing a letter to me than a composition for Verna; Mitch was certainly more concerned about impressing Andrea than Eileen.

•   •   •

The question, "What's in it for me?", is one both Daniel and Mitch implicitly ask as they learn to read and write. It is also the question practitioners implicitly, or explicitly, must ask when confronted by a new way of seeing the world, in this case, ethnographically. "What's in it for me?" is not the negative, selfish, cynical query it

may appear to be at first glance. Rather, it is the operative logical question all people tacitly ask as they make choices and decisions throughout their lives. As pointed out in the introduction, ethnographers assume that people act rationally to make sense of the world they experience; they choose their actions on the basis of what makes sense, "what's in it" for them.

That is why ethnography makes so much sense as a way of understanding and assessing literacy development. Seeing students' reading and writing as ways they have chosen to deal with their worlds helps practitioners realize that not only might degrees of intelligence or ability explain differences in literacy behavior, but differences in context might, too. If students cannot answer the question, "What's in it for me?" in some positive way, they have no reason to become literately different from the way they are, even if they have the ability to do just that.

Daniel and Mitch are cases in point. Clearly, both boys can understand what they read, can write at length, and can invest themselves in literacy activities. Why should they do so beyond the demands of the situations in which they find themselves? Both seem to have the necessary intelligence to standardize their language, their spelling, and their control of conventions, but why should they? Neither their schools nor their lives require such changes. It makes no sense for them to change from their perspectives at least; theirs are the perspectives that matter when literacy behavior is at issue.

Ethnography brings five questions to literacy assessment, questions that go beyond samples, tests, and scores to the context of literacy learning itself.

1. Is what the student has been taught important? What has he or she learned to value as personal qualities and markers of success? Does humility matter or saving face? Are passivity and conformity marks of a "good" student or do people need to stand out and distinguish themselves in any ways they can?

2. What has the student been taught to do socially? What kinds of social activities and relations has he or she learned to manage successfully? Only small group activities; only with people like himself or herself? Are different people and different settings perceived as "not mine" or as irrelevant or even dangerous?

3. What has the student been taught to do academically? What sorts of activities has the school provided? Drill and repetition? Worksheets and kits? Formulaic essays? Basal readers?

4. What has the student been taught is possible? What does he or she see as his or her future in life? Exactly what family members have always done? Exactly what peers are doing? Whatever he or she dreams for himself or herself?

5. What kinds of experiences has the child had? That is, has he or she consistently experienced learning as positive or negative?

Clearly, these questions cannot be answered through test scores, profiles, or through anything else a cumulative record may contain. These are questions of context, questions for ethnographic consideration, questions to help design literacy intervention and instruction. What students know about the world, what they believe is possible, what they consider useful and important, and how they have experienced learning and literacy in the past bears directly on how they will grow as literate individuals in the future. These factors also bear directly on how clinicians and teachers can help them become those individuals.

REFERENCES

Bissex, G. (1980). *GNYS AT WRK: A child learns to write and read.* Cambridge, MA: Harvard University Press.

Calkins, L. (1983). *Lessons from a child.* Portsmouth, NH: Heinemann.

Cazden, C., & John, V. (1971). Learning in American Indian children. In M. Wax, S. Diamond, & F. Gearing (Eds.), *Anthropological perspectives in education.* New York, NY: Basic Books.

Cole, M. (1981). *The zone of proximal development: Where culture and cognition create each other.* Unpublished manuscript.

Fishman, A. (1988). *Amish literacy: What and how it means.* Portsmouth, NH: Heinemann.

Heath, S.B. (1983). *Ways with words: Language, life, and work in communities and classrooms.* New York, NY: Cambridge University Press.

Mehan, H. (1979). *Learning lessons: Social organization in the classroom.* Cambridge, MA: Harvard University Press.

Michaels, S. (1983). Teacher/child collaboration as oral preparation for literacy. In B. Schieffelin (Ed.), *Acquiring literacy: Ethnographic perspectives.* Norwood, NJ: Ablex.

Mischler, E. (1979). Meaning in context: Is there any other kind? *Harvard Educational Review, 49,* 1–19.

Perl, S., & Wilson, N. (1986). *Through teachers' eyes: Portraits of writing teachers at work.* Portsmouth, NH: Heinemann.

Taylor, D., & Dorsey-Gaines, C. (1988). *Growing up literate: Learning from inner city families.* Portsmouth, NH: Heinemann.

Wagner, D. (1983). Rediscovering "rote": Some cognitive and pedagogical preliminaries. In S. Irvine & J.W. Berry (Eds.), *Human assessment and cultural factors.* New York, NY: Plenum.

Individual differences in script reports: Implications for language assessment

Barbara L. Ross, MS
PreDoctoral Fellow
Department of Psychology
University of Utah

Cynthia A. Berg, PhD
Assistant Professor
Department of Psychology
University of Utah
Salt Lake City, Utah

WHEN INDIVIDUALS are asked to describe routine events, their descriptions often exhibit characteristics of script reports (Schank & Abelson, 1977). A script has been defined as a set of expectations individuals have about routine events that is organized in a temporal-causal sequence of acts or single actions (Fivush, 1984; Nelson, Fivush, Hudson, & Lucariello, 1983). Individuals use the organization of scripts to describe routine events and to aid in their memory of specific instances of events (Bower, Black, & Turner, 1979). The organization of scripts has also been found to enhance children's use and comprehension of language (Constable, 1986; Furman & Walden, 1989; Lucariello, Kyratzis, & Engel, 1986). As a result of their facilitative organization, scripts have been used in language inter-

The research on which this article is based was supported by an NIMH PreDoctoral Fellowship awarded to Barbara L. Ross and was supported in part by a University of Utah Research Committee Faculty Grant awarded to Cynthia A. Berg.

Top Lang Disord, 1990,10(3),30–44
© 1990 Aspen Publishers, Inc.

vention techniques (Constable, 1986) and in formal and informal assessments of language that involve describing routine events, for example, Detroit Test of Learning Aptitude-2, Communicative Activities in Daily Living (Hammill 1985); making inferences about events, for example, Test of Language Competence (Wiig & Secord, 1985); and remembering script-related stories, for example, Clinical Evaluation of Language Fundamentals-Revised (CELF-R) (Semel, Wiig, & Secord, 1987).

Researchers who have examined children's script reports have suggested that scripts for routine events are very common across individuals, as scripts are based on common experiences (Nelson, 1981, 1986). However, the following script report from a 5-year-old girl who was asked to describe what happens when a person goes on an airplane trip illustrates that some idiosyncracies exist in script reports:

> You get money
> eat breakfast
> take a nap
> get in the plane
> sit down
> get lunch
> sleep all night
> wake up when it gets light out again
> get off the plane
> find a hotel

Although most of this child's description appears to be consistent with what we think of as a script for airplane travel, her comments about sleeping and waking are somewhat less traditional. We might conjecture that the child was confusing her description of what happens on an airplane trip with what ordinarily happens when she goes to sleep, which would account for the inclusion of the acts "sleep

all night" and "wake up [in the morning] when it gets light out again." However, after talking with her about her experiences with airplane travel, another explanation comes to mind. She reported that she had flown on an airplane many times and that all of her experiences flying involved trips from Utah to Argentina, South America, to visit her grandmother. Given this child's experience with international travel, it is reasonable that her script for airplane travel includes the acts "sleep all night" on the plane and "wake up when it gets light out again."

This child's script comes from our own work and illustrates how an individual's description of an event is related to his or her specific, yet typical, experiences. Other children in our study who did not have experience with international airplane travel did not include the act of "sleep all night" in their scripts. A common belief among script researchers is that idiosyncratic acts like "sleep all night" do not exist in well-formed scripts. In fact, such nontraditional acts have been referred to as distortions and deficiencies in script reports (Nelson, 1981). However, idiosyncracies occur frequently in the script reports of both children and adults and may be the norm, rather than the exception. We will argue that nontraditional acts are present in well-formed scripts to the extent that they are consistent with an individual's typical experience with the event.

The primary purpose of the article is to illustrate how individual differences in scripts may be found in verbal reports of everyday activities as well as memory for new events, such as those commonly used in language assessment. We will present the results of two studies that show that individual differences are extremely prevalent with respect to the number and content of acts included in script reports and that they impact memory for new script-related events. Implications of individual differences in script reports for language assessment will be discussed as script generation and script memory are commonly used in language assessment.

THE SCRIPT MODEL

The script model has been used to describe the way in which individuals come to understand and represent information about many routine events (Fivush, Hudson, & Nelson, 1984; Nelson, 1981). Two major features of scripts are wholeness and temporal-causal order. These two features may underlie the facilitative effect that scripts have in enhancing children's communicative abilities by providing an organized structure through which to communicate.

Wholeness

A script, like other forms of schematic representation, has been described as an "organized body of knowledge such that a part implies the whole and the whole is more than the sum of the parts" (Nelson & Gruendel, 1981, p. 138). In support of the idea that a part implies the whole, Schank and Abelson (1977) found that individuals often falsely recalled and recognized parts of a script that were not presented. For example, an individual presented with a list of actions for going on an airplane trip that includes packing and checking in at the gate is likely to report that other events involved in the airplane script were also presented, for example, getting a boarding pass, waiting for the plane, etc. In support of the idea that the whole is greater than the sum of its parts, researchers have found that the individuals apply what they know about one familiar event (airplane travel) to a novel, yet similar event (travel by train) (Schank & Abelson, 1977). The idea that the whole is greater than the sum of its parts is what Nelson and Gruendel (1981) described as the script's predictive power: Individuals use their experience with various events to understand events that they may never have directly experienced.

Temporal-causal structure

The temporal-causal structure of scripts is a feature that distinguishes scripts from other forms of schematic representation (e.g., scenes) (Nelson & Gruendel, 1986). Temporal-causal structure means that the order in which certain events occur in a script is constrained by other events in the script that precede and follow events either temporally (e.g., getting airplane tickets precedes getting on the airplane) or causally (e.g., picking up one's luggage follows only if you have checked in your baggage at the airport) (Nelson, 1984; Nelson et al., 1983). Research demonstrates that individuals of all ages, even very young children, have scripts that have temporal-causal organization. For

Research demonstrates that individuals of all ages, even very young children, have scripts that have temporal-causal organization.

example, when individuals are presented with scripted stories containing acts that do not conform to the typical temporal-causal structure of an event, children and adults reorder or exclude acts such that their recall corresponds with the typical temporal-causal structure of the events (Bower et al., 1979; Nelson et al., 1983).

The script characteristics that have been discussed, wholeness and temporal-causal structure, play an important role in how individuals understand and remember various activities. Although these characteristics seem to be present even in the script reports of young children, differences in script reports have been found across the life span.

SCRIPT DEVELOPMENT

Script generation

In contrast to research that characterizes children's memory as unorganized and fragmented, studies of children's scripts have found that even very young children remember routine events in a highly organized fashion (Nelson et al., 1983). The pervasive use of scripts even in early child development is illustrated by actions that Piaget (1967) characterized as examples of deferred imitation. Deferred imitations tend to be organized much like the events themselves, in a specified temporal-causal order. For example, young children who pretend to drive a car or shave their faces often proceed in a highly organized and accurate fashion consistent with the organization of scripts (Nelson, 1978). Research on script development has indicated that the scripts of young children are very similar to those of adults in

terms of their general structure and content, particularly when examining acts related to the primary goals of the script (e.g., flying for the event of airplane travel). Although there are data to suggest that even very young children have relatively well-organized scripts, there are some differences between the scripts of younger children and older children.

The scripts of younger children (ages 4 to 6 years) are characterized as being less detailed (Fivush & Slackman, 1986; Nelson, 1986; Slackman, Hudson, & Fivush, 1986) and shorter than those of older children and adults (McCartney & Nelson, 1981; Nelson & Gruendel, 1981). For example, Slackman et al. (1986) described three types of variable acts that elaborate and differentiate scripts that are rarely included in the scripts of young children but are present in the scripts of older children: (a) optional acts (e.g., "Sometimes you sleep on a plane"), (b) alternative acts (e.g., "You either look out the window or play cards"), and (c) conditional acts (e.g., "If the stewardess asks, you can go visit the pilot").

Even though script reports differ in their detail and elaboration as children develop, script reports are quite common across development and do not appear to contain idiosyncratic information (Fivush & Slackman, 1986; Nelson & Gruendel, 1981). For example, Nelson (1978) examined several script reports for three different scripted activities and found that only 4% of the acts were idiosyncratic (i.e., mentioned by only one child). Nelson and Gruendel (1986) also found extremely high consistency in the acts that were mentioned by 4-, 6-, and 8-year-old children. Although act consistency increased with age, even 4-year-olds mentioned the same acts on average 55% of the time.

Few studies have examined differences in script knowledge between late childhood and adulthood. However, some researchers have examined scripts during the adult life course. Light and Anderson (1983) found no age-related differences between younger and older adults in the general content and structure of scripts. They also found no age-related differences in the detail used to describe everyday activities or in the interindividual variability of scripts. Thus, research with adults indicates that scripts are also highly common across adulthood (Light & Anderson, 1983).

In summary, the literature on script development during childhood and adulthood points out many commonalities in the general structure and content of scripts throughout development. Although development in scripts occurs from early childhood to later childhood, research suggests that once developed, scripts are essentially the same for all individuals (Light & Anderson, 1983; Nelson, 1986). As scripts are considered to be well-developed by late childhood, idiosyncracies in script reports may be viewed as more deviant for older children than younger children and particularly abnormal for adults. However, the research that indicates that scripts are common across individuals uses methodological techniques that may account for much of the reported similarity in script reports.

Methodological issues in script generation

The assertion of commonality in script reports is so predominant that some defini-

tions even include the premise that scripts must be common because they are based on common experiences (Nelson, 1981). By positing that scripts are common across individuals, methodologies have been used that result in little variability in script reports. A brief consideration of methodological issues in script research will be presented to illustrate how the techniques used to elicit scripts may impact the degree to which idiosyncratic information is included in script reports. These methodological issues may be relevant for clinicians as the methods they use to elicit verbal reports may result in varying degrees of idiosyncracies in individuals' descriptions of events.

The methodological techniques used in script research that may have resulted in little variability in script reports involve the way in which scripts have been elicited from individuals and the selective use of certain types of script reports. These methodological techniques include selectively probing participants to elicit only common acts, explicitly instructing participants to report only common acts, and excluding acts or entire reports that are idiosyncratic. In a study of intersubject commonality in scripts, Nelson (1978) used extensive probing to elicit specific acts present in events, which she acknowledged may have ensured that many acts would be produced by most of the participants. Light and Anderson (1983) posed instructions to their participants emphasizing that "the task was to produce a list of common actions or events . . . that should not include idiosyncratic actions based on their own behavior but should list actions that would be typically performed by most people" (p. 437). In addition, each subject was instructed to produce approximately 20 actions, which undoubtedly constrained the number of acts that individuals reported, artificially shortening some reports and lengthening others. Furthermore, script reports were discarded that differed markedly from other reports in perspective. For instance, reports of a doctor's appointment that were given from the perspective of the doctor as opposed to the patient were not used in the study. As these methodological techniques may have inhibited the reporting of idiosyncratic information, it may be premature to conclude that there are no individual differences in script reports within any developmental level and few age differences in script organization between developmental levels. Our research (Ross & Berg, 1989) suggests that different methodological techniques for eliciting script reports may result in less commonality among the reports than has previously been found.

INDIVIDUAL DIFFERENCES IN SCRIPT REPORTS

The goal of our work with both children and adults has been to examine script reports using methods that do not discourage the reporting of idiosyncratic information. In two different studies, we asked individuals to describe commonly occurring events in sufficient detail so that another person would know exactly what the individual did during the event. As individuals related their scripts, they were probed to complete their descriptions with questions like "Does anything else happen?" until they responded "No." Individual differences in scripts were evaluated using two different measures: (a) an act consistency score and (b) the proportion of unique acts in a script. The act consistency score, previously used by Nelson (1986), is the percentage of individuals that mentioned a particular act. The proportion of unique acts, previously used by Light and Anderson (1983), is the proportion of acts mentioned by an individual that are idiosyncratic, that is, only mentioned by that one individual.

Preliminary work with children revealed that individual differences are prevalent in children's script reports. Ten 4-year-olds were asked to describe their scripts for airplane travel. The children were asked to describe what happens between the time they decide to go on an airplane trip and the time they leave the airport at their destination to a Mickey Mouse puppet who needed to follow their instructions. The children produced an average of 9.4 acts, with the number of acts ranging from 4 to 23. Only 6% of the acts were mentioned by more than half of the children in our study. Sixty-one percent of the acts were mentioned by only one child, a percentage much larger than the 4% found in the Nelson (1978) study described above. The proportion of unique acts mentioned by each individual ranged from 17% to 43%, with an average of 31%. These results suggest that individual differences are very prevalent in the script reports of young children.

A study was then conducted to examine the prevalence of individual differences in the script reports of adults (Ross, 1989; Ross & Berg, 1989). Thirty young adults (mean age = 22.9 years) and 30 older adults (mean age = 66.7 years) were asked to describe their scripts for airplane travel and doctor's appointments without limitations regarding the kinds or number of acts to produce. Each participant was asked to describe the events in two parts, to ensure that all participants had a similar understanding of the task. For the airplane script, participants were asked to describe what happens between the time they (a) decide to take an airplane trip and the time they are called to board the plane, and (b) between the time they are called to enter the plane and the time they leave the airport at their destination. For the doctor script, participants were asked to describe what happens between the time they (a) decide to see a doctor and the time they are called into the examination room, and (b) between the time they are called into the examination room and the time they leave the doctor's office. This division of events into two parts was the same for each individual and was based on pilot work that indicated that approximately half of the acts generated for these two events were included in each part.

Great variability in the number and kinds of acts that participants produced was found. The average number of acts generated for the airplane script was 28.1 and for the doctor script was 24.8. More importantly, the range of acts generated for both scripts indicated enormous variability in the number and kinds of acts produced (range = 12 to 62 for the airplane script; range = 12 to 78 for the doctor script). Several hundred different acts were generated to describe each half of the airplane and doctor script reports.

Act consistency scores were used to examine the degree of commonality in scripts. Mean act consistency scores were low for both the airplane script (an average of 1.7 and 2.0 people mentioned each

act for the first half and second half of the script, respectively) and the doctor script (an average of 1.8 and 1.2 people mentioned each act for the first half and second half of the script, respectively). Although great variability existed in the kinds of acts reported, some acts (e.g., packing, getting luggage) were mentioned by a majority of the participants.

The proportion of unique acts was used to examine the degree to which individuals included idiosyncratic acts in their script reports. Idiosyncratic information in the script reports ranged from 0% to 88% of the entire report, with an average of 30% for the airplane scripts and an average of 40% for the doctor scripts. Means, standard deviations, and ranges of proportion of unique acts by age and script type are presented in Table 1. These proportions indicate that a large percentage of the acts an individual generated in a script were mentioned by only one individual. There were significant age differences in the proportion of unique acts; older individuals had a higher proportion of unique acts than younger individuals. In addition, a higher proportion of unique acts was found for doctor scripts than for airplane scripts.

Table 1. Mean proportion of unique acts by age and story

	N	Mean	SD	Range
Airplane				
Young	30	.27	.14	.04–.56
Old	30	.33	.16	0–.62
Doctor				
Young	30	.35	.17	.10–.69
Old	30	.46	.20	.06–.88

Previous work has been based on the assumption that script reports do not contain idiosyncratic information; therefore, it may be suggested that the reports received from participants were not actually scripts. However, many of the characteristics used to describe and define scripts were found. For example, the reports describing airplane travel and doctor's appointments were consistently given in an appropriate temporal-causal sequence, preserving the temporal-causal order of the actual events. In addition, the majority of acts mentioned were given in the general, timeless form characteristic of script reports (Fivush et al., 1984) (e.g., "You board the plane" vs. "I boarded the plane"). The participants also indicated that their reports were based on their own experience with the scripted events, which is a characteristic of scripts first described by Schank and Abelson (1977). Therefore, we interpreted these reports to be script reports.

In summary, it appears that without methodological constraints, individual differences exist in the script reports of children and adults. Regardless of whether one looks at variability between acts or variability between individuals, our studies suggest that individuals do differ in the number and kind of acts included in script reports. The prevalence of individual differences in scripts appears to depend on the age of the individual generating the script and on the event being described. As script reports are often used in language assessments, it is important to acknowledge the extent of individual differences in typical script reports and when individual differences may be especially preva-

> *Regardless of whether one looks at variability between acts or variability between individuals, these studies suggest that individuals do differ in the number and kind of acts included in script reports.*

lent (e.g., for a particular scripted event or for a particular age group).

Given that individual differences do occur in the script reports of both children and adults, it is necessary to begin to understand the origin of these differences. Examining the loci of individual differences in script reports will be particularly important as clinicians attempt to determine whether idiosyncracies in verbal reports used to assess language are due to variations in experience, mental maturity, or language ability. The original work of Schank and Abelson (1977) and the results of our work suggest that individual differences in script reports may result from variations in experience.

THE ROLE OF EXPERIENCE IN PRODUCING INDIVIDUAL DIFFERENCES IN SCRIPTS

Schank and Abelson (1977) suggested that individuals differ in their perception and interpretation of events and that these perceptions may significantly affect their script representation for various events. One element of perspective that Schank and Abelson offer to account for individual differences in script development involves the individual's role in the event.

For example, a pilot and a passenger, due to their different roles in airplane travel, are likely to have very different perspectives of the event that may contribute to differences in their script for this event. A pilot might mention acts such as "Check flight instruments" and "Clear for take-off," whereas a passenger would not. Other aspects of personal perspective mentioned by Schank and Abelson include differences in goals (flying to save time vs. to acquire frequent flyer mileage), habits (doing paperwork on the plane vs. playing games), motivation (flying out of necessity vs. flying for pleasure), affectivity (being anxious about flying vs. being very comfortable), and involvement (directly experiencing airplane travel vs. reading about it).

In addition, Schank and Abelson posit that differences in the amount and kind of experience with an event affect the development of personal scripts. Frequent exposure to obstacles or exceptions with an event may make idiosyncratic events become part of an individual's script for that event. For example, an individual who consistently misses flight connections may include acts such as "Arrange for a new flight" or "Arrange for accommodations near the airport," whereas someone who had never missed flight connections would not be likely to include such acts in his or her airplane script.

Nelson and Gruendel (1986) also proposed that some features of experience (frequency of occurrence, centrality to the child, and affect) have an impact on script development. However, they posited that these factors are the same in degree for children of the same age, thus equating age and experience. For instance, they asserted that the event of going to a birthday party is low in frequency, high in centrality, and high in affectivity for all young children. Although this work addresses how scripts may vary across different events (e.g., birthday party vs. going to a restaurant), it does not address how scripts for a single event may vary across individuals. According to the original work of Schank and Abelson (1977), however, all of these factors are highly dependent on both the specific experiences and personal characteristics of the individual involved in the event. Rather than using these factors to assess the development of scripts for different events in the same children, it may be more useful to use these factors to support the possibility that more personalized scripts develop with varied experience across children.

The confounding of age and experience has created reluctance among researchers to examine differences in experience and knowledge at one particular age. By using age as the sole measure of experience, Nelson and Gruendel (1986) and others have assumed that as children get older, they acquire more knowledge about the world as well as about routine events. Although this assumption may often be true, Chi (1978) and others (Chiesi, Spilich, & Voss, 1979) have found that younger individuals may possess greater knowledge in specific domains than older individuals. Chi's work and others' (see Chi & Ceci, 1987, for a review) support the notion that knowledge or expertise, rather than age, is often the critical factor affecting memory. By equating age and experience, researchers seem to make an additional assumption that amount of experience is the critical factor affecting script development as opposed to other elements of experience (e.g., specific content). Research has shown (Chi & Ceci, 1987) that experience contains many facets (specific content, structure and organization, amount) and that each of these facets may play a role in script development. Our own research (Ross, 1989; Ross & Berg, 1989) suggests that specific experience is more critical in producing individual differences in scripts than the global amount of experience a person has with an event.

In our study of individual differences in adults' scripts, we examined many features of experience with airplane travel and doctor's appointments. We assessed individuals' experience with these events via a questionnaire that included questions regarding the number of times an individual had participated in the events, the types of different experience they had with the events (types of flights and types of doctors), when they last experienced the events, their attitudes toward the events, etc. Despite great ranges in the amount of experience participants had with airplane travel (range = 2 to 999 trips during lifetime) and doctor's appointments (range = 0 to 600 visits during lifetime), no strong relationships between amount of experience and our measures of individual differences in script reports were found. In other words, there were no strong and consistent relationships between several "amount of experience" factors (e.g., the number of times an individual had participated in an event) and the total number of acts or the proportion of unique acts individuals included in their scripts.

Rather, it appeared that the specific content of a person's experience with an event was the critical factor in producing individual differences in scripts. As stated earlier, there were large variations in the kinds of acts reported by subjects regarding the same scripted event that appeared to result from individuals' specific experience with these events. Evidence for this assertion comes from ratings that individuals provided of their own script report regarding how typical the acts were in their experience. Both younger and older adults rated the acts in their script as typical to very typical (5.3 on a 6-point scale). Even acts that were mentioned by only one participant and seemed quite atypical were rated by that participant as being typical in their own experience: "You find out if there's road construction"; "You see if there are any famous people on the plane"; "You make a trip to the airport the day before the flight to check the timing." Although the results of our study suggest that the specific content of an individual's experience with an event is critical in producing individual differences in script reports, other possibilities exist. As it is difficult for individuals to estimate accurately the amount of experience they have with frequently occurring events such as airplane travel and doctor's appointments, amount of experience should be considered in future research.

Regardless of whether it is the amount or specific content of experience that is critical in producing individual differences in script reports, it appears that some aspect of experience is key. Many studies on the constructive theory of memory (e.g., Bartlett, 1932) have hypothesized that individuals use their own experiences as a basis for remembering new events and stories about such events. A second component of our study involved examining the impact of individual differences in script reports on recall and recognition of new script-related stories, as is required in some forms of language assessment.

THE IMPACT OF INDIVIDUAL DIFFERENCES ON MEMORY FOR NEW SCRIPT-RELATED STORIES

Previous research on the impact of knowledge and experience on script memory suggests that individuals of all ages remember events in terms of their expectations about an event rather than the actual event (Bower et al., 1979; McCartney & Nelson, 1981; Nelson et al., 1983). Individuals rely so strongly on their expectations or scripts for events that they are virtually unable to recall or describe individual instances of an event independently of their script. As our results suggest that individuals differ in the content of their scripts, individuals may not be using similar scripts for events to guide their memory for new events. Older adults exhibited larger individual differences in their script reports than younger adults, as may be the case for young children and older children, and the impact of this differential heterogeneity on memory was examined.

In our study of individual differences in adults (Ross, 1989; Ross & Berg, 1989), we hypothesized that an individual's personal script for an event is critical for memory of new stories, not some generic script that all individuals hold in common. To test our hypothesis, we tailored script-related stories to be either very similar to or

different from each subject's own script for two different events. The high similarity stories contained 12 acts that were generated by the participant and 4 new acts. The low similarity stories contained 4 acts generated by the participant and 12 new acts. We anticipated that when an individual was presented with a script-related story that was substantially different from that individual's script, she or he would make more errors in attempting to remember the story than if that story were similar to her or his script.

We found that individuals recalled significantly more acts from the stories that were highly consistent with their own script than from the stories that were very different from their own script (recalled 46% of the acts for high consistency stories and 32% for low consistency stories). In addition, individuals made more errors in the recall of stories that were less similar to their own personal scripts. These errors made the stories conform more to their own personal script by the addition of acts from their personal script. Subjects correctly recognized acts that were presented in the highly similar stories significantly more often than in the stories that were less similar to their own scripts. In addition, more acts were falsely recognized for stories that were less similar to their own scripts than for stories that were more similar. Overall, the subjects' memory for stories that were very similar to their own scripts was more accurate than for stories that were very different from their own scripts.

In summary, these results suggest that individual differences in script reports have a strong influence on memory for new information. As scripts have also been

> *Overall, the subjects' memory for stories that were very similar to their own scripts was more accurate than for stories that were very different from their own scripts.*

shown to have an impact on the comprehension and use of language (e.g., Constable, 1986), individual differences in scripts may affect these language processes and thus performance on tests of linguistic abilities.

THE IMPACT OF INDIVIDUAL DIFFERENCES IN SCRIPT REPORTS ON LANGUAGE ASSESSMENT

Research on memory and language development suggests that the comprehension of language and quality and quantity of information conveyed through language are strongly influenced by the knowledge individuals possess (Klatzky, 1980; Schank & Abelson, 1977). Recently, the script model has been used to examine this relationship between knowledge and linguistic abilities. Several studies have shown that the temporal-causal organization of scripts enables children to use and comprehend language more effectively than in less organized contexts (Constable, 1986; Furman & Walden, 1989; Lucariello et al., 1986; Shatz, 1983). In script contexts, children use more semantically complex language (e.g., speak significantly more often of past and future events, speak of many different topics in one conversation) and are better able to

answer questions than in other contexts (Furman & Walden, 1989; Lucariello et al., 1986).

One explanation for the facilitative effect of scripts on language use and comprehension is that scripts may lighten the load of other cognitive demands enabling children to use more advanced linguistic skills (Shatz, in Lucariello et al. 1986). Knowledge of familiar situations may allow children to concentrate on language as opposed to being distracted by generating content on an unfamiliar topic. This facilitative effect of scripts is consistent with the research on memory, which shows that children's memory is more organized for script-related events, particularly for familiar events, than for other types of events (Nelson et al., 1983). Although this work illustrates how greater knowledge can aid memory and language, it may also be that knowledge impedes individuals' performance if their previous knowledge is inconsistent with the demands being placed on them (Chi & Ceci, 1987; Ross, 1989). That is, individuals who possess knowledge that is inconsistent with the information surrounding a linguistic task may perform more poorly than individuals who possess more consistent knowledge. This potential detrimental effect of knowledge becomes a concern in the interpretation of some language assessment tests.

The results from our studies indicate that experience and knowledge about events produce great variability in the scripts people generate for routine events. In addition, these individual differences in scripts have an impact on memory for new script-related stories. Our results have direct implications for two different kinds of language assessment techniques: (a) spontaneous or elicited language samples that involve describing routine activities, and (b) tests or informal tasks assessing language comprehension that involve memory for events.

Current assessment of language production involves informal and formal evaluations of descriptions of events. Informally, clinicians frequently engage a child in a conversation and elicit information about highly scripted events such as what happened during the child's school day, a holiday, or a family vacation. They may then examine the description for the number and kinds of acts mentioned, sequencing of acts, relations between the acts, specificity of the description, off-topic remarks, and other aspects of the narratives.

This kind of analysis is presently used in the Story Construction subtest of the Detroit Test of Learning Aptitude-2 (Hammill, 1985). In this subtest, children are asked to tell a story that describes a picture of an activity that may be highly scripted (e.g., a basketball game). One criterion used for scoring the children's stories involves assessing their ability to sequence acts within a story, a critical aspect of script reports. Depending on the amount and kind of experience children have with such events, their ability to sequence "appropriate" acts with regard to such events may be hampered.

Scripted events are also used to assess the linguistic capabilities of adults. For example, the test of Communicative Activities in Daily Living (CADL) requires individuals to use their knowledge of familiar events in order to role-play and answer questions about a visit to the doctor's office, grocery shopping, and driving a car (Holland, 1980). As our research indicates, individual differences in experience with such routine events may influence descriptions that are generated for the events in several ways: length of description, kinds of acts mentioned, and ability to describe "appropriate" or "common" acts for the events. Imagine two individuals, one who has no previous experience with going to a doctor's appointment versus an individual with extensive and varied experience. We would expect these two individuals to differ in their descriptions of the event in terms of length, kind, and idiosyncracy of the acts mentioned. Because of the way in which many language assessment tools are evaluated, individuals with shorter, less detailed, and more idiosyncratic descriptions of these events may score lower on these tests. Such performances may not reflect poor language skills, but rather a different perspective of the event (or the task) and varied experiences with the event. Only through further examination of individuals' specific experience with events will clinicians understand the source of some poor language samples.

Individual differences in scripts may also influence language assessments that require making inferences about commonly occurring events. For instance, the Making Inferences Subtest of the Test of Language Competence (Wiig & Secord, 1985) requires children to make inferences about highly scripted events such as going to a restaurant, a birthday party, and a movie. If children make incorrect inferences, they are then asked to relate their experiences with the event in the extension testing section. If the child's experience is "reasonable" or "plausible," then the child is retested on the inferences subtest. The manner in which the retest is scored, however, does not relate the child's experience with the event to his or her performance. Nevertheless, relating a child's specific experience with events such as going to a restaurant may be critical in accurately assessing whether performance on the inferences subtest is related to the child's experience or to a language deficit. That is, a child's idiosyncratic experience could lead to his or her making an inference that is inaccurate given the elements of the problem, but is accurate based on the child's own experience.

Finally, individual differences in scripts may influence language evaluations that involve assessments requiring individuals to remember a script-related story. One section of the CELF-R (Wiig et al., 1987) requires individuals to listen to stories and answer questions about their content. For example, some of the stories involve events such as preparing for a Halloween party, entering a high school science fair, and working out family differences. If individuals taking this test had experiences with these events that differed in specific content from the stories, their memory of the stories may be impeded in favor of their experiences. For instance, an individual who had entered numerous science fairs might have an extensive script for entering such fairs and might easily impose his or her personal script onto the story he or she was asked to remember. An individual with little or no experience with entering science fairs would not be at such a disadvantage. Again, performance on these tests may reflect differences in knowledge or experience, in addition to differences in linguistic abilities.

In summary, individual differences in script reports may have an impact on performance in many language assessments, particularly those that use descriptions of routine events as the basis for the assessment. Based on our work, certain age groups may be at a particular disadvantage relative to other age groups in their knowledge of routine events and thus may perform poorly in assessments that require knowledge of routine events. In addition, the nature of the events used in language assessments must be considered as certain events may involve more or less variability in the acts comprising them.

• • •

Individual differences in script reports are found when methods are used that do not discourage or eliminate the reporting of idiosyncratic acts. Individual differences in script reports are important, and they may require a reevaluation of much of the work on scripted events including how scripts impact adults' memory for new script-related events.

Clinicians should carefully examine language assessment procedures that require the client to relate a story about a particular event and to remember a new event. Differential experiences with such events may result in impoverished or elaborate scripts of them and may result in the imposition of such scripts on new script-related events. An impoverished language sample may result as much from a lack of experience with the event used to generate the language sample as from a linguistic deficit.

Individual differences in script reports can no longer be neglected. Although individual differences greatly complicate work on scripts such that we can no longer speak of a "generic" script that all individuals possess, such work may better approximate the scripts that individuals follow in their daily lives for routine events.

REFERENCES

Bartlett, F.C. (1932). *Remembering: A study in experimental and social psychology.* Cambridge, England: Cambridge University Press.

Bower, G.H., Black, J.B., & Turner, T.J. (1979). Scripts in memory for text. *Cognitive Psychology, 11,* 177–220.

Chi, M.T.H. (1978). Knowledge structures and memory development. In R.S. Siegler (Ed.), *Children's thinking: What develops?* Hillsdale, NJ: Erlbaum.

Chi, M., & Ceci, S. (1987). Content knowledge in memory development. *Advances in Child Development and Behavior, 20,* 91–143.

Chiesi, H., Spilich, G., & Voss, J. (1979). Acquisition of domain-related information in relation to high and low domain knowledge. *Journal of Verbal Learning and Verbal Behavior, 18,* 257–273.

Constable, C.M. (1986). The application of scripts in the organization of language intervention contexts. *Event Knowledge, 10,* 205–230.

Fivush, R. (1984). Learning about school: The development of kindergartners' school scripts. *Child Development, 55,* 1697–1709.

Fivush, R., Hudson, J., & Nelson, K. (1984). Children's long-term memory for a novel event: An exploratory study. *Merrill-Palmer Quarterly, 30,* 303–316.

Fivush, R., & Slackman, E. (1986). The acquisition and development of scripts. In K. Nelson (Ed.), *Event knowledge: Structure and function in development.* Hillsdale, NJ: Erlbaum.

Furman, L.N., & Walden, T.A. (1989, April). *The effect of script knowledge on children's communicative interactions.* Paper presented at the meeting of the Society for Research in Child Development, Kansas City, MO.

Hammill, D.D. (1985). *Detroit tests of learning aptitude.* Austin, TX: PRO-ED.

Holland, A. (1980). *Communicative abilities in daily living: A test of functional communication for aphasic adults.* Baltimore, MD: University Park Press.

Klatzky, R.L. (1980). *Human memory: Structures and processes* (2nd ed.). San Francisco, CA: W.H. Freeman.

Light, L., & Anderson, P. (1983). Memory for scripts in young and older adults. *Memory & Cognition, 11,* 435–444.

Lucariello, J., Kyratzis, A., & Engel, S. (1986). Event representations, context, and language. *Event Knowledge, 7,* 136–160.

McCartney, K.A., & Nelson, K. (1981). Children's use of scripts in story recall. *Discourse Processes, 4,* 59–70.

Nelson, K. (1978). How young children represent knowledge in their world in and out of language. In R.S. Seigler (Ed.), *Children's thinking: What develops?* Hillsdale, NJ: Erlbaum.

Nelson, K. (1981). Social cognition in a script framework. In J.H. Flavell & L. Ross (Eds.), *Social cognitive development: Frontier and possible futures.* New York, NY: Cambridge University Press.

Nelson, K. (1984). The transition from infant to child memory. In M. Moscovitz (Ed.), *Advances in the study of communication and affect* (Vol. 10. Infant memory). New York, NY: Plenum.

Nelson, K. (Ed.). (1986). *Event knowledge: Structure and function in development.* Hillsdale, NJ: Erlbaum.

Nelson, K., Fivush, R., Hudson, J., & Lucariello, J. (1983). Scripts and the development of memory. In M.T.H. Chi (Ed.), *Contributions to human development: Trends in memory development research* (Vol. 9). New York, NY: Karger.

Nelson, K., & Gruendel, J. (1981). Generalized event representations: Basic building blocks of cognitive development. In M.E. Lamb & A.L. Brown (Eds.), *Advances in developmental psychology* (Vol. 1). Hillsdale, NJ: Erlbaum.

Nelson, K., & Gruendel, J. (1986). Children's scripts. In K. Nelson (Ed.), *Event knowledge: Structure and function in development.* Hillsdale, NJ: Erlbaum.

Piaget, J. (1967). *Six psychology studies.* (D. Elkind, Ed.). New York, NY: Random House.

Ross, B.L. (1989). *The impact of individual differences in scripts memory for script-related stories.* Unpublished master's thesis, University of Utah, Salt Lake City, UT.

Ross, B.L., & Berg, C.A. (1989). *The use of personal scripts in remembering new events across adulthood.* Paper presented at the meeting of the Society for Research in Child Development, Kansas City, MO.

Schank, R.C., & Abelson, R. (1977). *Scripts, plans, goals, and understanding.* Hillsdale, NJ: Erlbaum.

Semel, E., Wiig, E., & Secord, W. (1987). *Clinical Evaluation of Language Fundamentals—Revised.* Austin, TX: Psychological Corporation.

Shatz, M. (1983). Communication. In P.M. Mussen (Series Ed.), J.H. Flavell & E.M. Markman (Vol. Eds.), *Handbook of child psychology* (Vol. 3). New York, NY: Wiley.

Slackman, E., Hudson, J., & Fivush, R. (1986). Actions, actors, links, and goals: The structure of children's event representations. In K. Nelson (Ed.), *Event knowledge: Structure and function in development.* Hillsdale, NJ: Erlbaum.

Wiig, E.H., & Secord, W. (1985). *Test of language competence.* Columbus, OH: Charles E. Merrill.

Progress in language and literacy learning: Ongoing assessment in the classroom

Elaine R. Silliman, PhD.
Professor
Department of Communication Sciences
  and Disorders
University of South Florida
Tampa, Florida

Louise Cherry Wilkinson, EdD
Professor and Dean
Graduate School of Education
Rutgers, State University of New Jersey
New Brunswick, New Jersey

Lauren P. Hoffman, MAT
Assistant Director
Program Planning and Development
South Metropolitan Association
Flossmoor, Illinois

THE VALIDITY OF a plan for assessment of children's language and literacy knowledge is determined in large part by the philosophy, principles, and practices that guide learning and teaching. As Gardner (1991) notes, "One can have the best assessment imaginable, but unless the accompanying curriculum is of quality, the assessment has no use. It will simply sit on a shelf, unused and unusable" (p. 254).

In this article, we describe the development and implementation of an observationally based plan to assess the language and literacy skills of students with severe language learning disabilities. This observational plan is specifically directed to the authentic assessment of children's progress in learning language and literacy skills within the classroom. Developed collaboratively by speech-language pathologists (SLPs), teachers, administrators, and investigators, the plan has been implemented as an integral part of the special education program

We gratefully acknowledge the assistance of Christi Wujek, Assistant Supervisor, and Sue Workman, Supervisor, both of the Communication Development Program, for their significant contributions to and support of the work described in this article.

Note: Extracts of this article appear in Documenting authentic progress in language and literacy learning: collaborative assessment in classrooms, *Topics in Language Disorders* 1993;14(1), 58–71.

for students with severe language learning disabilities who attend a public school.

A first step in the development of a plan for authentic assessment is to understand clearly the relationship between a program's philosophy and its educational/intervention principles and practices (Gardner, 1991). The following section describes these connections for the Communication Development Program (for a more detailed description of the program, see Hoffman [1990] and Silliman & Wilkinson [1991]).

PROGRAM

The Communication Development (CD) Program, initially established in 1978, is an educational program of the South Metropolitan Association (SMA), a cooperative association of 55 school districts located in Illinois (South Cook County and North Will County). The purpose of SMA is to provide special education services for children and adolescents with low-incidence disabilities, including severe communication disorders.

The CD Program consists of five educational levels: lower primary (comparable to a combined kindergarten and first grade), primary, intermediate (comparable to a combined fifth and sixth grade), middle school, and high school (grades 9 to 12). At the high school level, instruction is departmentalized.

PHILOSOPHY AND PRINCIPLES

The philosophy of the program is based on the belief that communication processes unite teaching and learning. Listening, speaking, reading, writing, and spelling are interrelated communicative processes that emerge from and are nurtured by social collaboration with teachers, parents, and peers. This philosophy also recognizes that a language learning disability is a chronic condition that significantly influences all areas of cognitive, linguistic-communicative, and social development.

Several principles emerge from this perspective. First, the goal of instruction is to enable communicative competence; hence the focus of teaching and learning is supporting students' abilities through the facilitation of active learning-how-to-learn strategies across mediums of communication. Second, an active approach to learning depends on how adequately students understand the purposes, relevance, and applications of what is being learned. Third, the focus of instruction is facilitating transitions from oral to literate uses of communication; students should progress from being primarily oral style communicators to being more capable users of literate styles of communication in both spoken and written domains. Fourth, the aim of a communication process approach is to "assist students in functioning in environments that are the least restrictive given their needs, abilities, and the academic contexts in which they are required to function" (Hoffman, 1990, p. 85).

PRACTICES

Collaboration and transdisciplinary teams

The instructional staff involved in the program work as a transdisciplinary team. Teams consist of a SLP certified by the American Speech-Language-Hearing Association who also is a classroom teacher; an educator of the deaf (selected because of the background in language and speech development); a school social worker; a career educator; and a teaching assistant. Efforts are made to include family members as part of the team.

In implementing communication goals for each student, team members cross traditional disciplinary boundaries in their planning, assessment, and instruction. Each is also committed to professional growth. Because the program's philosophy is directed toward understanding the entire student, all disciplines and their perspectives are valued on the team; team members approach problem solving and decision making within a collaborative framework. Attention is given to supporting and nurturing teams by the team members themselves and by the administration.

Instruction

Instruction for the students in the CD Program is designed to build on students' strengths through integrating language and literacy activities across all content areas. In addition, the development of metacognitive and metalinguistic strategies is incorporated into all units, which are theme guided. Depending on students' needs, each unit may take from 5 to 8 weeks to complete.

For example, during the 1991–1992 school year, students in the lower primary level participated in six theme-based units: a fairy tale unit, a sea unit, a dinosaur unit, a jobs unit, a foods unit, and a circus unit. At the intermediate level, units consisted of an art history unit, a magic unit, and a human body unit. At the high school (grade 10) level, the year's English course consisted of units on the production of a television news show, the relevance of good literature (*Tom Sawyer*) to teenage lives, and vacation planning. Students are partners in theme implementation; therefore, two important objec-

tives of theme-based learning are to support students in becoming active decision makers and to help them be more explicitly aware of their own strengths, talents, and needs.

Educational climate

The educational climate in the CD Program is one in which innovation is valued and change is accepted. The program is characterized by continual self-assessment, including an external evaluation every 3 years. As part of programmatic self-assessment, the expectation has been that the educational staff would continue their professional commitment to finding more effective ways for improving students' learning.

During the process of designing change, however, the staff came to two conclusions: The previous traditional plan for assessing effectiveness failed to relate assessment procedures to instructional goals and procedures, and too much time was spent on assessment tasks that yielded limited amounts of useful information. Because the need for change was the result of a bottom-up process of staff decision making, the staff were ready to shift to the authentic assessment of students' progress.

THREE ESSENTIAL COMPONENTS FOR IMPLEMENTATION

The assessment plan was developed for students who demonstrated significant language learning difficulties and who were placed in a special program in a public school. A comparable plan can be implemented in any setting along the educational continuum, however, as long as the conditions for implementation are created and appropriate personnel, training, and time are provided. A major issue for plan implementation is consistency across staff in their approach to authentic assessment. To enhance consistency, three components were identified as essential.

Developing a common frame of reference for assessing students' progress

One of the staff's first needs was to understand more adequately the background rationale for the use of observationally based assessment of progress. The operating premise was that an assessment plan should be theory driven to achieve the integration of teaching and learning. Otherwise, the danger would exist for assessment to be reduced to a set of techniques that remain unconnected to a unifying conceptual framework (Silliman & Wilkinson, in press-a, in press-b). The central principles motivating the plan for authentic assessment derived from neo-Vygotskian theory: In both developmental and educational arenas, effective teaching is seen as assisted performance (Gallimore & Tharp, 1990):

At the outset, the child and adult work together, with the adult doing most of the work and serving as an expert model. As the child acquires some degree of skill, the adult cedes the child responsibility for part of the job and does less of the work. Gradually, the child takes more of the initiative, and the adult serves primarily to provide support and help when the child experiences problems. Eventually, the child internalizes the initially joint activities and becomes capable of carrying them out independently. (Campione & Brown, 1987, p. 83)

In short, effective teaching consists of collaboration through the support of discourse and the progressive transfer of responsibility from the adult to the child for managing his or her own learning. The adult's role is primarily that of a facilitator who engages children in instructional conversations as the means for assisting them in their successful progress along a continuum from novice to expert.

Determining whether changes in a student's patterns of performance are authentic is often difficult (Howell & Morehead, 1987; Wilkinson & Silliman, in press). At least four reasons may account for this difficulty:

1. Not every change is meaningful.
2. Initially, change may consist of less visible "flickers" rather than obvious behaviors.
3. Change is not invariably continuous or linear; rather, its course may be more like a series of peaks and valleys (Bain & Dollaghan, 1991).
4. As previously noted, the assessment of students' progress needs to be guided by a theory if teaching and learning are to be integrated (Silliman & Wilkinson, in press-a, in press-b).

During the 1990–1991 school year, staff, administrators, and university consultants met in a series of inservice meetings to develop consensus on theoretical orientations and principles. A follow-up planning committee consisting of team members from the various educational levels, the diagnostic team, and the CD Program supervisor consolidated a common frame of reference. From the beginning, two points were agreed upon. First, an authentic assessment plan would serve as both an educational and a research document. Second, because team members were also the actual teaching staff, they could assume a unique position as participant observers of their own classrooms. As a result of what they actually did with students, team members would be able to describe from within their own perspectives how "knowledge can be generated, challenged, and evaluated . . . and how their own interpretations of classroom events are shaped" (Lytle & Cochran-Smith, 1992, p. 452).

In the summer of 1991, the planning group drafted an authentic assessment plan, incorporating feedback from team members and the university consultants. The 1991–1992 school year was to serve as the pilot year for the plan.

Providing professional support for risk taking

A shift in the way that assessments are carried out requires risk taking by all team members. To support risk taking, the CD staff needed to communicate. They needed to share their observations and expectations with each other and to be provided with appropriate material and technical resources to begin the process of assessing students within classroom settings.

For example, videotaping was an essential part of the assessment plan. Each team was required to videotape at least three times during a unit. For most of the team members, classroom videotaping was a new experience that involved the learning of new skills in a public medium. In addition, each team provided adequate back-up material for each unit, from diagnostic and program planning information to evaluative information about changes observed in the students and in themselves as teachers. Table 1 presents the checklist developed to assist team members in the gathering of comparable information for each unit and to help them with some procedural issues connected with videotaping.

In addition to collaboration among the staff, the staff and administration maintained systematic and ongoing collaboration with the university consultants throughout the planning and pilot years. For example, during the pilot year (1991–1992), university consultants met with staff and administration three times: before initiating the formal plan in the classroom, at midyear, and at the end of the school year. Procedural and substantive issues and concerns were discussed. Videotapes from units were reviewed as a group. Workable formats were developed to organize and analyze the information being collected. Revisions were made in procedures and processes as appropriate.

The collaboration among staff, administrators, and investigators promoted the positive and productive sharing of expertise and enhanced mutual awareness of teaching goals and strategies (Silliman & Wilkinson, 1991). As a result, the staff became their own agents of change in a relatively rapid period of time.

Allowing flexible time management

One additional issue confronting the CD staff was how best to manage the time of team members. This issue needed ongoing attention and support from the administration. The staff required time to experiment with and to understand new observational systems and tools. The experience of working on a transdisciplinary team, where ongoing collaboration and support of team members' needs were essential elements for success, appeared to be critical for addressing time management issues. Transdisciplinary team experience also seemed to be equally critical for implementing the assessment procedures.

Table 1. Educational staff checklist for data collection

Videotaping mechanics	Diagnostic and program planning information	Accompanying documents	Videotaping content and process	Evaluative information
See target students? Hear target students? Camera on before and after lesson?	IEP goals and objectives included? Updated goals, objectives, and strategies included? Portfolio documents dated? Copies of "stickies" (Post-it Note summaries)?	Daily class schedule? Classroom map? Description of unit? Description of lesson videotaped? Schedule for lesson? Copies of unit back-up material, including books, charts, graphs, etc.? Documents dated?	Opportunities provided for target students to participate? Target students included in discussion or pulled into discussion? Task appropriate for target students?	Document changes via personal diary, videotape, or audiotape three times per unit. Include: • Date _____ • Name _____ • Educational level _____ Summarize: • What are the most important changes you have observed about: 1. the instructional process 2. the target students 3. yourself • Other comments

THE STUDENTS AND EDUCATIONAL TEAMS

The students

The educational staff and program administrators selected eight students, two each from four educational levels, to be followed during the pilot year. Table 2 presents the characteristics of the participating students, their distribution across the educational levels, and the team composition for each student dyad. Junior high level students were not included for the pilot year.

Student selection was based on several factors: typicality of the overall student population, including the lack of other complicating conditions such as hearing loss or multiple handicaps; an equal distribution of boys and girls across the educational levels; the diversity in socioeconomic and ethnic backgrounds; and parental agreement to participate in the assessment activity. Complete diagnostic and individualized educational program (IEP) information was available for each of the eight students (in keeping with P.L. 94-142 requirements and special education regulations of the Illinois Board of Education). The kinds of traditional assessment information available included speech and language reports, educational reports, social development reports, psychological reports, and, for the high school students, reports on vocational skills.

The educational teams

The educational teams differed in their experience as teachers and in the duration of their working on classroom teams. The years of experience ranged from 3 years (two SLPs at the lower primary and primary levels) to 10 years (an educator at the intermediate level). In terms of team experience, the 1991–1992 school year was the first for which the two SLPs at the primary level had been teamed together. Although content areas at the high school were departmentalized, the high school staff was teamed as a single unit to coordinate educational planning for all the high school students. The SLP and career educator participating in the pilot year study had been part of this planning team for 5 years.

THE FRAMEWORK FOR AUTHENTIC ASSESSMENT

The assessment plan was aimed at providing a longitudinal record of students' progress through developing in-depth case studies for individual students (Fujiki & Brinton, 1991). Traditional case studies often result in a snapshot of a student's current level of performance because assessment is performed at a single point in time (McTear & Conti-Ramsden, 1992). In contrast, the CD approach reflects a qualitative form of a repeated sampling design where the eight students served as their own controls. Each case study evolved from the continuous sampling and interpretation of multiple sources of information within the real communicative contexts of the classroom. Thus a major goal is to document the transition from novice to expert, or how and in what ways individual students are assisted to move from current levels of competence to new levels of competence. The belief is that, in the long term, this design will be sufficiently robust to address two interrelated intervention issues: effectiveness (i.e., does an intervention program work) and, most critically, efficacy (i.e., how and why does an intervention program work; Silliman & Wilkinson, in press-b).

Table 2. Students and teams selected for observational assessment of progress (1991–1992)

Student[a]	Level[b]	Birth date	Sex	Ethnic background	Date enrolled in CD Program	Total students in whole class	Team
Clayton	LP	8/08/85	M	African American	August 1991	7	1 SLP
Jamie	LP	11/06/84	F	White	August 1991		
Abbey	P	12/29/83	F	White	August 1990	16	2 SLPs
Charles	P	12/09/83	M	White	August 1990		
Alice	I	7/25/81	F	White	January 1989	15	SLP and educator
Irwin	I	12/17/83	M	Hispanic	October 1991		
David[c]	HS (grade 9)	6/07/77	M	African American	August 1990	29 in high school program, 11 in career education class,	Career educator
Jackie[c]	HS (grade 10)	8/06/75	F	African American	August 1983	8 in English class	1 SLP

[a] Names have been changed to protect confidentiality.
[b] Educational levels:
LP, lower primary (preprimary); P, primary; I, intermediate (upper primary); HS, high school.
[c] Jackie's assessment occurred in her developmental English class; David's was conducted in his career education class.

KEY COMMUNICATIVE PROCESSES

Figure 1 displays the three communicative processes that were the focus of the plan for the observationally based assessment. These three processes influence each other.

The inner circle depicts the social organization of teaching and learning. This organization is built and orchestrated by the ways SLPs and teachers use language to achieve the goals of language and literacy learning. Questions of interest for assessment purposes were (1) how activity structures worked to facilitate the integration of educational and communicative goals for target students as individuals and as group members and (2) the nature and appropriateness of discourse scaffolding strategies and patterns used by team members in a facilitative role. This communicative process was considered important for addressing issues of intervention efficacy. In this instance, efficacy was defined as explanations of how and why a communication process approach works (or does not work) to achieve authentic changes in language, learning, and development.

The social organization of learning influences and is influenced by the advances individual students make in learning how to learn, the second process. The basic issue to address is the effectiveness of strategy use by target students within and across activity structures and content areas. A key component involves how and in what ways students at various educational levels learn to monitor and evaluate their communicative strengths and needs and, as a result, select appropriate strategies to achieve their goals.

Effectiveness of intervention is a major aspect of efficacy. It is the aspect most often addressed in the research literature (Kavale, 1990). The largest circle represents effectiveness as a continual transition from novice to expert learning along the multiple levels of the oral-literate continuum. The critical issue involves whether observed changes are authentic advancements, which are defined as more effective and consistent demonstrations of the transfer of responsibility for learning from the teacher to the student (Silliman & Wilkinson, in press-b). Within specific content areas, evidence that students can take on more responsibility for their own learning should be interconnected with greater use of effective strategies and less need for discourse support from teachers.

OBSERVATIONAL TOOLS FOR ASSESSMENT

The box titled "Types of Observational Tools" summarizes three kinds of observational tools that were included in the assessment plan: categorical, narrative, and descriptive. These tools were intended to

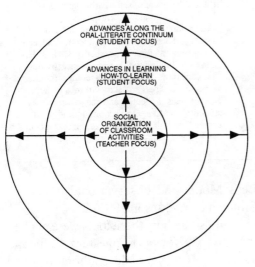

Figure 1. Key communicative processes.

Types of Observational Tools Used in the Assessment of Authentic Progress

Categorical (closed systems)
- Rating scales and checklists
  1. Student assessments: Used within and across content areas for ongoing self-assessment on changes observed in abilities and needs
     —Self-profiles (easy and hard subject content)
     —Learning style questionnaires (self-awareness)
     —Unit evaluations (ease and difficulty of task demands and learning strategies)
- Classification systems: Teacher/investigator assessments
  1. Scaffolding profiles: Categories of scaffolding (high, medium, low) into which student discourse needs are classified
  2. Specific categories of analysis applied to oral discourse (teacher–student(s), student–student, etc.): Used to document the specific kinds and amounts of discourse support necessary to achieve successful outcomes (see also descriptive tools, below)
  3. Specific categories of analysis applied to student-generated works-in-progress (logs, journals, stories, drawings, reports, newspaper articles, graphs, dictionary collections, etc., all of which can make up a portfolio collection): Used to document specific strategy development and scope of its application across written text structures (see also descriptive tools, below)

Narrative (open systems)
- Teacher assessments
  1. Anecdotal notes (on-line daily observations of targeted behaviors, implemented by a Post-it Note chart in each classroom): Used within and across content areas to record significant behaviors as they actually occur in relation to individual student goals
  2. Assignment notebooks: Used to summarize progress within a skill area over time
  3. Quarterly progress notes: Directed to families as a summary of progress within a unit for individual students
  4. Student-generated works-in-progress (see categorical tools, above, for examples and purpose)

  5. End-of-unit assessments: Conducted at the end of each unit to document the nature, scope, and creativity of strategies that students display for integrating their educational and communication goals (students typically choose how they want to demonstrate what has been learned during the unit)
  6. Teacher self-assessment of instruction: Used at the end of each unit to analyze and summarize what has been learned about the effectiveness of instructional strategies and any necessary modifications
- Teacher/investigator assessments
  1. Running records (written chronological accounts of a specific activity; for example, any classroom activity, including end-of-unit assessments, based on the videotape of that activity): For educational purposes, each educational team prepares a minimum of three during the school year to relate the structure and goals of activities to intended outcomes for individual students; for research purposes, running records are constructed for each of the three videotapings of each unit
  2. Critical incidents (written accounts derived from running records of significant interactional patterns): Address in finer detail a key event or events emerging from a running record

Descriptive (open systems)
- Teacher assessments
  1. Classroom maps (classroom arrangement of specific activities): Used to show the physical arrangement of the classroom, including student–teacher locations, for particular activities
- Teacher/investigator assessments
  1. Transcriptions of teacher–student and student–student oral discourse: Used to identify and analyze specific patterns of teacher or student discourse scaffolding within and across activities
  2. Transcriptions of written discourse (student works-in-progress): Used within and across content areas to identify and analyze changes in students' written expression, including discourse functions, text structures, linguistic complexity, and spelling

---

capture different aspects of the three key communicative processes at different levels of detail. Also, each general type of tool has advantages and disadvantages connected with its use, which are not discussed here (for a complete review of the Observational Lens Model and observational tools, see Silliman & Wilkinson 1991).

To illustrate how these tools were applied initially, we focus on one target student, Jackie, a $16^{1}/_{2}$-year-old sophomore level student.

Jackie entered the CD Program when she was 8 years old and had received intensive language-based instruction within a small group classroom setting since that time. At age 4 years, she was language delayed; her mother described her as reluctant to talk. This reluctant talker descriptor still remained relevant for Jackie as an oral communicator at age 16½ years.

According to the formal triannual evaluation conducted in January 1992, Jackie had progressed but still displayed significant academic problems in language arts, math, and general knowledge. She functioned from 2 to 5 years below age level on standardized measures of oral language comprehension and production and reading comprehension. Her word recognition skills for both reading and spelling, however, were at or above grade level. The speech-language reevaluation reported that Jackie continued to struggle with planning and problem solving, including effectively managing her participation in various forms of oral discourse. She was still a reluctant talker. It appeared that the rapidly shifting demands of oral discourse processing created stress for her and subsequent withdrawal from participation.

The SLP's assessment of Jackie's strengths and needs was as follows:

- Oral discourse
  1. Can manage conversational interaction with peers or highly familiar adults.
  2. When conversational partners are less familiar or when academic language use is required, has difficulties with effective strategies for rapid information retrieval, maintaining topical continuity over more than three to five turns, and repairing comprehension breakdowns.
  3. When unable to continue a conversation, does not maintain normal eye gaze, and will often stand silently or walk away.
- Written discourse
  1. Has basic skill in reading, writing, and spelling.
  2. Prefers print as a means of communication, possibly because it allows her more time to engage in advance discourse planning.
  3. Peers view her as a good reader and speller and use her as a resource for these purposes.
- Cooperative problem solving
  1. When assigned role of leader in cooperative learning projects, can obtain input from team members, provide encouraging comments, or recommend an appropriate strategy to a peer.
  2. In the role of team leader, however, continues to need high levels of teacher support to generate alternative solutions to a problem or to carry out multiple steps.
  3. When not a team leader, becomes a passive participant.

Jackie's assessment of her strengths and needs was as follows:

- Oral discourse
  1. Listening and speaking are difficult
- Written discourse
  1. Writing and reading are strengths.
  2. Certain learning strategies help my reading, such as repeating information to myself, noting key words, and underlining main points.
- Cooperative problem solving
  1. Have confidence about my ability to think.

2. Have less confidence about my
   ability to stop being impulsive
   while working through a problem.

During the period from November 1991 through February 1992, which overlapped the triannual evaluation, Jackie and her classmates were engaged in a cooperative learning project in her developmental English class. This project involved the actual production of a television news show, and Jackie was the director; she was responsible for writing the script, among other jobs. The SLP was also the English teacher. Her overall goal for Jackie during this unit was as follows: Jackie will apply her learning strategies to social and linguistic problem solving by recognizing her strengths in reading and writing, utilizing these strengths to facilitate her comprehension and composing of expository discourse (e.g., the script), and assuming increased responsibility for obtaining, retaining, clarifying, and evaluating linguistic information. The documentation issue concerned how adequately this goal related to the specific activities of the unit and the outcomes for Jackie.

Categorical tools

The box titled "Types of Observational Tools" presents information about categorical tools, which are closed systems for observation; that is, they have preset categories into which all behaviors or events are coded. A wide range of behaviors typically serves as the focus of assessment, and the coded categories can be summed in some manner to describe the observation quantitatively.

Checklists and rating scales

Checklists and rating scales are top-down tools because observed behaviors are fit into predetermined categories. Their content typically extends over a broad range of classroom activities and behaviors. Moreover, assessment is often after the fact. Because assessment takes place after a learning activity has concluded, it is retrospective and primarily oriented to outcomes.

The box titled "Types of Observational Tools" lists examples of checklists and rating scales. These were included in the assessment plan for two major purposes. One was to provide the opportunity for students to participate in assessment through obtaining self-evaluations of advances made over time in three areas: **various content areas**, through rating the ease or difficulty of learning over time (e.g., in speech, language, math, reading, art, or music); **awareness of learning styles and strategies** (e.g., identifying how they learn best and when, where, why, how, and with whom they learn their most difficult subject best [Larson & McKinley, 1987]); and **judgments about the task demands and strategies specific to particular thematic units** (unit evaluations).

For example, upon completing the television production unit (February 25, 1992) Jackie, along with her peers, was asked to rate each of 10 situations along a 5-point scale (1, "very hard for you to do"; 5, "easy for you to do"). She gave a rating of 3 (sometimes easy and sometimes hard) to four situations: taking notes on this unit, bringing everything you need to class; understanding the articles you read by yourself, and completing your job for the news show. A rating of 5 was given to the remaining 6 situations: keeping your folders organized, vocabulary words, homework assignments, understanding the articles we read in class, writing in your journal, and working in your project/peer groups. Each student was also asked to choose one example of each rating and to justify it. Jackie rated vocabulary words as 5 ("They are easy to understand") and understanding the articles she read on her own as 3 ("because some of the words are easy but when it comes to the harder words I have to ask a teacher").

A second purpose for the use of categorical tools involved the teacher's assessment of general behaviors over time. For example, quarterly progress notes, a narrative tool, could be reconstructed as a rating scale to reflect the student's progress at the end of a theme in areas such as learning new vocabulary specific to the theme and changes in reading, writing/spelling, listening/speaking, and math skills.

The wide view generated by checklists and rating scales does not allow specific patterns to emerge. Because these categories are often global and not always clearly related to each other, observers must often engage in a high degree of inferencing about whether the behavior fits the category. Jackie's ratings of certain situations illustrate this point. Her judgments were valuable because her perspective was being offered on general aspects of the learning process. How these individual self-evaluations reflect specific patterns is unclear, however. For example, consider the following question about Jackie's acquisition of new word meanings: What is the relationship between her evaluation of easy in understanding the vocabulary words in the unit and the variability she alluded to in understanding some of these same meanings when reading them on her own?

It should be noted that the assessment plan contained flexible choices about the se-

lection of checklists and rating scales available commercially or generated by the staff in house. With the exception of the student evaluations, choices had to be adapted to the developmental and educational levels of the students.

Classification systems

Classification systems are bottom-up tools that allow greater detail to be seen (see the box, "Types of Observational Tools"). They are tailored for analyzing specific patterns of behaviors that emerge from observation rather than being superimposed on the observation itself. Classification systems work best when a low degree of inference is required for categorizing. They are most appropriate when the observer sees a close relationship between behavior as it actually occurs in a particular context and the unit of analysis selected to examine that behavior.

In the assessment plan, these systems allowed the teacher or investigator to examine a particular discourse ability as it advanced along the oral-literate discourse continuum. For example, changes in student-generated dialog journals could be tracked according to the features of the developmental phases outlined by Westby and Costlow (1991), from premessage awareness through the self-generation of several words to the development of the written narrative.

When the degree of detail is fine within the classification system, however, even more refined tools are needed. For example, the assessment of a student's need for scaffolding may be directed to the effectiveness of intervention. Scaffolding profiles also involved teachers' assessments. These profiles were initially developed as a means for documenting the level of discourse assistance necessary for individual students to be successful within particular tasks across activities. A high level of discourse scaffolding would occur when the teacher needs to assume full responsibility for successful participation by providing the student with a specific strategy. A medium level of scaffolding occurs when the teacher needs only to provide specific cues (prompts) that would then lead the student to draw on a best fit strategy to be successful. A low level of discourse scaffolding occurs when the student independently or with minimal cues uses appropriate strategies. Low-level scaffolding could also be defined as the teacher acting as a mentor, giving help only when the student requested. These discourse scaffolding profiles were also to be completed for all students every 4 months.

A greater level of detail is needed when the purpose becomes highly specific. One example pertains to examining the specific discourse scaffolding strategies that teams use to guide students in learning how to integrate and apply connections among what they know, what they want to know, how to find out what they want to know, and how to express their new understandings through a variety of communication modes, including speech and print (Westby & Costlow, 1991). In this situation, the focus of observation is oriented to the how and why question of intervention. How are discourse processes working (or not working) for individual students in assisting them to accomplish personally selected communication goals?

Narrative tools

Narrative tools are open systems for observing. Open systems may also contain predetermined categories, but unlike categorical tools the categories are not mutually exclusive, and multiple avenues can be available for assessment. Moreover, open systems can be modified, added to, or subtracted from as observations are collected and attempts are made to analyze them.

Narrative tools are selected when the purpose is to record broad segments of events or behaviors that occur in the classroom. In general, these tools consist of systematic and detailed written descriptions of what a student does, says, or writes. One advantage of narrative tools is that they can provide permanent longitudinal documentation of student progress.

The box titled "Types of Observational Tools" also summarizes the major categories of narrative tools included in the assessment plan and the level of detail allowed by each type. The narrative tools used by teaching teams varied, but all used anecdotal notes daily and weekly, portfolio collections routinely, quarterly self-assessments of changes observed in the instructional process for both the target students and themselves as teachers (see Table 1), and running records and critical incidents. Running records were constructed from the videotaping of the three sessions from each unit; preparation of critical incidents from the running records was an optional decision.

Anecdotal notes

This narrative tool records on-line observations of student behaviors that are a focus for assessment. If the degree of detail provided is general in description, then only a broad view results. In a broad view, relationships are not seen among goals, the activities to support these goals, and the actual outcomes.

**Post-it Note Chart and Examples of the SLP's On-Line Observations
during the Television Production Unit**

2-4-92
Jackie assisted another student with editing the TV script. Did a nice job helping student identify What didn't sound right. She also provided appropriate suggestions for revisions.

2-5-92
Jackie asked for help on her typing assignment. She needed assistance with calculating the tabs and margins.

2-6-92
Jackie reported that she talked to student (WG) about interviewing her again for the TV script since she had lost the original information. Set up interview on her own! Good problem solving.

2-1-92
Observed Jackie providing good encouraging comments during group practice. She said I think you can be louder a bit and your eye contact is good.

2-14-92
When a peer mentioned that he did not have money to buy valentines, Jackie suggested, You can always make one. She also used a visual/gestural cue to encourage the same peer to look up (at the camera) during practice videotaping.

2-18-92
Jackie showed a new student how to write the days date when he wrote in his journal.

If the degree of detail is specific to particular behaviors that are instructional/intervention goals, however, then over time anecdotal notes should reveal relationships that are consistent with a moderate level of detail. A sample of on-line observations (anecdotal notes) about Jackie's strategy choices, as written by her high school SLP/teacher and two of her peers, illustrates this moderate level of detail (see the boxes titled "Post-it Note Chart" and "Examples of Post-it Notes").

**Examples of Post-it Notes Written by Jackie's Peers
during the Television Production Unit**

2-1-92
Helped me practice told me to be louder. CC

2-7-92
Helped me set up the camera when it wasn't her job. RN

The procedure followed for collecting and compiling these observations involved using Post-it Notes. A weekly Post-it Note chart was displayed in each classroom, where it was easily accessible to both students and staff. Once an observation was recorded with the date and the student's name, either the student or the teacher could post the observation on the chart. At the end of each week, the educational team summarized the observations collected for each student in a computer file. This summary was then placed in the student's portfolio. If an observation was a negative description, it was recorded and included in the weekly summary but not displayed on the classroom chart.

Team members needed experience in writing behaviorally focused observations to meet the purposes of this tool. In other words, clearly focused observations were the product of explicit understanding of goals for individual students.

Portfolio collections

The assessment plan contained a detailed description of portfolios. A portfolio collection is not simply a file that holds a student's work. It has been defined as:

A purposeful collection of student work that exhibits the student's efforts, progress, and achievements in one or more areas. The collections must include student participation in selecting contents, the criteria for selection, the criteria for judging merit, and evidence of student self-reflection. (Paulson, Paulson, & Meyer, 1991, p. 60)

Decisions about the content of portfolios were based on specific criteria, including collaboration with the student, a schedule for collecting and evaluating information, a process for gathering samples across content areas of a student's ideas, revisions of those ideas, and finished work. The portfolio was located where it would be readily accessible to the student and teacher. Examples of materials included in a collection are logs of books read by students or parents; stories written by a student or class; writing journals and dialog journals; letters written to different audiences; specific examples of strategies learned; student reports, drawings, or number writing; student self-assessment scales; and videotapes or audiotapes demonstrating what had been learned.

Because a portfolio is a continuous collection of students' work, at the end of the school year the educational team and student reviewed together which portfolio contents best exemplified what had been learned. This process of joint decision making resulted in identifying which aspects of the file were to constitute the student's permanent file. The file contained monthly evaluations of progress as reflected through portfolio content to identify instructional modifications. For example, Jackie spontaneously decided to write to one of the authors after she completed the television unit (see the box, "Jackie's Letter"). This letter revealed a more integrated perspective, in comparison to the rating scale cited previously, of what she had learned from the unit about how to communicate, the meaning of that learning, and how the experience affected her.

Running records and critical incidents

Running records are a written account of a specific activity. They provide a systematic, intensive, and chronological record in everyday language of the complete stream of behavior as it actually unfolds.

Jackie's Letter (All Spelling, Punctuation, and Spacings Retained)

2-27-92

Dear Dr Silliman
   I am studying about T.V. jobs in English class and I was
nominated as the director because I am an organizing person,
get along well with people and I like to be a director someday.
We were working on a news show and I was an anchorwoman I had
to write scripts about different topics in school. I had to
think about different ideas for the news show. I had interview
people, some of the stories I reported were on the new books in
the library and the people who made the honor roll. I had to
practice and memorize it until I get it right, I also had to
rehearse it for many weeks. I had some strategies I used when I
was working on my script. I somebody helped me on my script I
was down some notes when I interview a person. I got to run a
video camera I liked it allot. When we video taping for the
news show it was hard because nobody wanted to look in the
camera we were embarrassed. I know I was. it was hard for me to
talk and looked in the camera at the same time. After we finished video taping we got to watch the tape was good eye contact, good posture, speaking loud and clearly and about how
fast they were speaking. When we were first working on this
unit it was harder than I thought because we had a lot of work
to do. When I was working in groups it was hard because sometimes hard to get along with people.
   We got started on Tom Sawyer we each have a book about him.
We took notes on it, and we are getting ready to make our story
chart. I hope you enjoy the tapes.

From
Jackie

In constructing running records from the videotaped lessons, team members did not select or evaluate what they thought was important, Rather, the purpose of running records was to allow observers, educational team members, program administrators, and the university consultants to develop a joint frame of reference for the particular activity. From the running record, it became possible to understand the structure of the activity and its goals; how this structure unfolded over time through different phases and tasks; expectations for how students were to participate as individuals and as group members, including the target student; and how participants sustained interaction and repaired breakdowns in communication.

The box titled "Excerpts" gives samples taken from the running record on the planning of a television news show to be produced by students in the sophomore level developmental English class. The 49-

---

Excerpts from the Running Record on the Planning of the Television News Production (November 21, 1991; Time Elapsed in the Session Is Indicated at the Left)

3:00–9:30

Jackie chooses a question from the Knowledge Cup and orally reads: "What is one thing you've learned about TV since we started this unit?" T [teacher] repeats the question. Approximately 22 seconds pass without Jackie responding. T asks Jackie if there is a problem followed by another 15 seconds of silence on Jackie's part. T comments about the amount of time that has passed and reminds Jackie of a strategy she could use for obtaining extra time. Another 20 seconds of silence follows and T asks Jackie if she understands the question. Jackie says that she does but cannot remember. T encourages Chad and Ralph to assist Jackie in strategy selection. Both suggest, with some support from T, that Jackie use her notes, look at the learning board, or ask a question to recall the information. With guidance from T, Jackie eventually refers to her notes and identifies *TV Guide* as a resource for finding out what television shows will be on.

13:00–26:55

The purpose of the investigation plan is introduced. T reviews the members of the planning committee and the three "C's" of committee work: Cooperation, Communication, and Cuing. Next, questions for the committee to review are reread and T asks about possible resources that can be used to answer the questions. Students make suggestions for calling, writing, or visiting a television studio and, after discussion, decide that writing a letter would be best. The library is also suggested as a resource, which, then, leads to discussion of key words that might be used to build a card catalogue about TV production.

26:56–35:05

T asks the group to identify another resource. Ralph suggests that they ask the teacher from the TV studio in the school. They are then helped to spell the teacher's name. Next, each student chooses a committee assignment based on how they view their abilities. Jackie says she will call the school TV studio because she is a good listener; Chad states that he will write a letter to a local television station because he is a good writer; and Ralph says he will go to the library because he likes the library and is a good researcher.

---

minute, 29-second session, which occurred on November 21, 1991, focused on two aspects: what students had learned about television and video production through the use of "Knowledge Cup" questions, and what they needed to know to write an investigation plan. Participants included the SLP/teacher and three students: Jackie (the target student), Ralph, and Chad.

Running records are not inherently longitudinal documentation. As the excerpts in the box show, they are oriented to preserving a specific period of time and context. To obtain the kind of big picture afforded by a running record, team members needed experience with how to focus on and synthesize the basic elements of a running record and how to avoid the writing of evaluative statements in preparing the written narrative. A second step in obtaining a complete big picture involves the reconciliation of conflicting perspectives on the events that transpired or the sequence in which events took place. This is an essential step because groups of observers select and interpret information differently. All members of the planning team, including program administrators and the university consultants, participated in this reconciliation process for the videotapes and accompanying running records by independently reviewing each one.

Running records allow observers to see the communicative context of a single activity at a moderate level of detail. Critical incidents, in comparison, provide a closer view of that context. They are used to obtain a relatively small amount of detailed information in narrative form to address a specific question of interest arising from the running record. For example, with the SLP/teacher present in the classroom, Jackie's typical style of interaction was nonassertive, including peer interaction. She did not routinely initiate topics or contribute new information unless prompted to do so. This pattern occurred particularly when the activity was one in which she had to engage in more linguistically explicit oral exchanges about her content knowledge (e.g.,

the first segment from the Knowledge Cup running record, where Jackie is asked to specify one thing she learned about television since the unit began).

A different view of Jackie emerged from the running record of December 9, 1991, however. During this session, which involved assignment of jobs for the television news show, the SLP/teacher was called out of the classroom but inadvertently left the video camera running. The incident, shown in the box titled "Critical Incident," began when the teacher left the room and ended 2 minutes, 35 seconds later, when she returned. Participants included Jackie and two other female classmates, Samantha and Gerry. Chad was also present. All three girls were friends.

With the SLP/teacher absent from the room, Jackie and her female peers immediately shifted to and sustained a more oral style of speaking. This style shift showed

---

Critical Incident: Jackie's Change in Discourse Style and Affect
(December 9, 1991; Duration: 2 minutes, 35 seconds)

Jackie, Samantha, and Gerry remain in their seats; they are seen and heard to giggle. Chad sits with his head down writing in his notebook. Jackie introduces the topic of a car bought by a female friend all three girls know (but whose name is never mentioned). She is visibly animated, smiling and gesturing as she tells of the four-door car whose back doors did not work and how one had to climb over the front seat to get to the back. All three girls laugh as Samantha says that Jackie bumped her head three or four times and Jackie responds with "Child, I coulda bumped my head three or four times." The conversation continues with much laughter when Jackie states that she thought that the car would be a sharp one, but that she kept hitting her head to get out of the car. Gerry contrasts this car with another friend's car where the doors work. Jackie reiterates she thought it would be a sharp car but that it was all dirty. Samantha then shifts the topic to the store they all went to where she bought some earrings and a tape that, together, cost about 14 dollars. Jackie then shades the topic and elaborates on her going to the record store with Samantha, purchasing a tape that cost $21.35, then finding she did not have enough money, and having to ask Samantha if she had a dollar or a quarter. All three are laughing when T [teacher] reenters the room. Immediately, the three girls alter their posture and their affect. The incident ends when T asks "How's it coming (their assignment)?"

Jackie to be an assertive contributor, capable of relatively sophisticated topic management with her peers without any breakdowns in retrieval. At the same time, this style shift simultaneously signaled Jackie's equal status and solidarity with her peers (Rees & Gerber, 1992).

The detailed level of information obtained from the critical incident shows how moment-to-moment changes in students' interpretation of their conversational roles influence their choice of discourse styles, including linguistic choices made about message construction, as well as the speed and automaticity of their information retrieval. These interpretations subsequently affect the big picture obtained of a student at any particular point in time.

Descriptive tools

In the assessment plan, the selection of descriptive tools, such as transcription of critical incidents, was a choice for the teams. When the purpose of assessment involves the documentation of a developing communicative process across situations, however, then more refined levels of analysis are required to see patterns in detail. How the aspects of particular information are classified (analyzed) determines the level of detail that emerges from assessment.

In Jackie's case, an important aim of assessment during the television production unit was to document changes in her ability to engage more independently in social and linguistic problem solving in cooperative learning. Students were given assignments to interview school staff and other students. Before "going out into the real world," they generated questions to ask and practiced interviewing each other. Jackie was hesitant to conduct actual interviews, afraid that she would make a mistake. She created numerous reasons for not having completed the interviews and script on time, such as, "I left it [the script] at home" and "I forgot it, so I can't do it," and she was the last to complete the assignment. Her peers convinced her to finish her work, encouraging her about the importance of her role to the project's completion. Thus the process of learning over time how to draft, edit, and revise different kinds of expository discourse, such as the script for the television news show (see the box titled "Jackie's First and Final Draft"), could provide the communicative context for an assessment of effectiveness. Units of analysis could include productivity as measured in T-units, the complexity of subordination strategies, and the extent to which writing became more integrative through the use of more diverse cohesive devices (Scott, 1989).

In contrast, when the purpose of Jackie's assessment was to provide detail on the scope and stability of specific developments that were occurring in the transfer of responsibility, then the most detailed level of analysis was needed. A fine-grained classification system for examining specific aspects of classroom discourse was the most appropriate tool for analysis. Questions to ask included how and in what ways the discourse strategies of the SLP/teacher supported Jackie's progressive internalization of planning strategies across modes of expression (oral or print), discourse structures (narrative or expository), and communicative functions (e.g., creating an autobiography or creating a television script). In this situation, efficacy issues—the how and why of intervention—motivated assessment.

Jackie's First and Final Drafts of Her Television News Show Script (All Spellings, Punctuations, and Spacings Retained)

First draft

Benton High School has received new books in library some examples are: Chicago Fire Disneyland: inside story, Suicide. They are very interesting books to read. You can go down to the library and check it out.

In woodshop Chad is making bows and varnish them. They are making cups and varnish them, making shelves, and making a wooden or metal tool boxes, and making clocks, a key rack. Also making a maple spoon, a step stool, and wood ducks. He use plan sheets, write down the measurements of what size the material has to be, if he has a problem his instructor give him a strategy to lay out the wood and see how many inches to cut it. The class is fun also you can make projects youn never made before. The tests are hard you have study very hard., take notes of everything the instructor writes down. They have to know how to use the tools, wear safety glasses in woodshop.

In the future, there will be some new books, teach the class how to use first aid in case of an emergency.

Wymona G has made the honor roll during the 1st semester. She has gotten all A's and B's in some of her classes, there is a list of the people who made the honor roll. There are ways to get on the honor roll, they are: Honors with distinction All A's, High Honors All A's except one B, Honors All A's and B's.

Final typed version (typed in uppercase)

WYMONA G MADE THE HONOR ROLL DURING THE 1ST SEMESTER. SHE HAS GOTTEN ALL A'S AND B'S IN HER CLASSES. THERE IS A LIST OF POEPLE WHO MADE THE HONOR ROLL IN THE MAIN LOBBY. THERE ARE THREE WAYS TO GET ON THE HONOR ROLL:
1.) HONORS WITH DISTINCTION - ALL A'S.
2.) HIGH HONORS - AA A'S EXCEPT ONE B.
3.) HONORS - ALL A'S AND B'S.
WORK HARD AND GET GOOD GRADES AND YOU TOO COULD BE ON THE HONOR ROLL.

BENTON HIGH SCHOOL HAS RECEIVED MANY NEW BOOK IN THE LIBRARY THIS YEAR. SOME OF THE BOOKS INCLUDE: THE CHICAGO FIRE; DISNEYLAND: THE INSIDE STORY; AND SUICIDE. THEY ARE INTERESTING BOOKS TO READ. YOU CAN GO DOWN TO THE LIBRARY AND CHECK THEM OUT.

I RECENTLY HAD THE OPPORTUNITY TO INTERVIEW CHAD C ABOUT HIS WOODSHOP CLASS. IN WOODSHOP, CHAD IS MAKING BOWS AND VARNISHING THEM. THEY ARE MAKING CUPS, SHLEVES, CLOCKS, KEY RACKS AND THEY ARE VARNISHING THEM. THEY MAY ALSO MAKE WOODEN OR METAL TOOL BOXES. CHAD HAS ALSO MADE A STEP STOOL, MAPLE SPOON, AND WOOD DUCKS. HE USED PLAN SHEETS, WROTE DOWN MEASUREMENT OF WHAT SIZE HIS MATERIALS HAD TO BE. CHAD SAID THAT IF HE HAD A PROBLEM, HIS INSTRUCTOR GAVE HIM A STRATEGY TO LAY OUT THE WOOD AND SEE HOW MANY INCHES TO CUT IT. HE SAID THE CLASS IS FUN AND YOU CAN MAKE PROJECTS YOU NEVER MADE BEFORE. HE TAKES NOTES OF EVERYTHING THE INSTRUCTOR WRITES DOWN. IN HIS CLASS, HE HAS TO KNOW HOW TO USE THE TOOLS, AND WEAR SAFETY GOGGLES. IN THE FUTURE, HE WILL GET A NEW BOOK AND LEARN HOW TO USE FIRST AID INCASE OF AN EMERGENCY. THIS SOUNDS LIKE A FUN CLASS SO KEEP IT IN MIND IF YOU NEED AN ELECTIVE CLASS.

EFFECTS OF CLASSROOM-BASED ASSESSMENT ON TEACHING AND LEARNING

The process of developing and implementing the assessment plan described here had a number of effects, both intended and unexpected, on the educational teams, students, and program.

Intended effects

The educational teams articulated significant professional growth during the pilot year as a result of plan implementation and their new roles as participant observers. Although the time required for implementation remained an issue, it appeared that the benefits of the information obtained outweighed the negative effects associated with increased commitment of time. Collaboration among team members became more focused, areas were identified more readily for additional inservice, and changes were designated in the formulation of instructional goals and objectives as team members came to understand students in new ways.

For example, it became apparent that, across educational levels, the actual focus of students' instruction, including Jackie's instruction, was often inconsistent with their written goals and objectives. A new tool, the Assessment and Instructional Profile (AIP), was developed in response to this finding. The AIP, implemented for the 1992–1993 school year, is an interim step in the use of a more integrated and flexible format for the IEP. The intent is for educational teams to use this tool to connect and monitor goals, objectives, scaffolding needs, and outcomes in a more systematic way.

Because the CD Program is supported by 55 school districts, it became critical that this constituency understand and accept the new process for measuring students' progress. Effort was continuously expended over the pilot school year to involve the special education representatives from the sending school districts in the new assessment plan. At the annual review meeting held at the end of the 1991–1992 school year, these representatives completed a survey on the nature and quality of the information that emerged; they unanimously indicated their approval.

Unexpected effects

As the assessment plan evolved, numerous unexpected effects also emerged. The Post-it Notes procedure for documenting on-line observations increased the staff's emphasis on students' strengths. Significantly, this assessment procedure increased student collaboration with peers and with the teaching staff. Across educational levels, students began to observe when one of their peers engaged in a behavior meriting the posting of a "sticky" (e.g., see the box titled "Examples of Post-it Notes"). Parents of target students also began to use Post-it Notes at home and to send them to school when their children demonstrated communicative strategies that were developmental and instructional priorities.

Videotaping served to increase the staff's understanding of their personal teaching style, including awareness of how their teaching discourse was or was not consistent with a facilitative role. Videotaping combined with the preparation of running records also increased collaboration among the educational teams on unit and lesson planning. Moreover, videotaping became a self-evaluation tool for Jackie, who discovered that she enjoyed being on camera. She began to analyze her presentation of self, which appeared to be a significant step in her social and emotional development.

At the level of the program, the plan had an impact on the basic process of assessment for determining students' eligibility and needs for special services. This assessment process was altered as a result. Finally, at the institutional level, the concept of the assessment plan was deemed appropriate for other educational programs in the SMA agency. A study group was created to assist all educational programs in providing more meaningful and authentic assessment for all students.

• • •

A collaborative assessment plan designed to examine the effectiveness and efficacy of a communication process approach is not a static entity. It involves more than adding a few new techniques to an existing assessment repertoire. Rather, it requires understanding the intricate relationship among philosophy, principles, and practices. It challenges us to think of assessment as an integrated, continuous, and natural part of the everyday activities of the classroom because any teaching–learning interaction contains potential assessment information. In the broadest sense of its meaning, authentic assessment should be approached as a dynamic, evolving, social process jointly constructed over time through the multiple perspectives of students, their families, educational staff, administrators, and investigators.

REFERENCES

Bain, B.A., & Dollaghan, C.A. (1991). The notion of clinically significant change. *Language, Speech, and Hearing Services in Schools, 22,* 264–270.

Campione, J.C., & Brown, A.L. (1987). Linking dynamic assessment with school achievement. In C.S. Lidz (Ed.), *Dynamic assessment: An interactional approach to evaluating learning potential* (pp. 82–115). New York, NY: Guilford.

Fujiki, M., & Brinton, B. (1991). The verbal noncommunicator: A case study. *Language, Speech, and Hearing Services in Schools, 22,* 322–333.

Gardner, H. (1991). *The unschooled mind: How children think and how schools should teach.* New York, NY: Basic Books.

Gallimore, R., & Tharp, R. (1990). Teaching mind in society: Teaching, schooling, and literate discourse. In L.C. Moll (Eds.), *Vygotsky and education: Instructional implications and applications of sociohistorical psychology* (pp. 175–205). New York, NY: Cambridge University Press.

Hoffman, L.P. (1990). The development of literacy in a school-based program. *Topics in Language Disorders, 10* (2), 81–92.

Howell, K.W., & Morehead, M.K. (1987). *Curriculum-based evaluation for special and remedial education.* Columbus, OH: Merrill.

Kavale, K.A. (1990). Variances and verities in learning disabilities intervention. In T.E. Scruggs & B.Y.L. Wong (Eds.), *Intervention research in learning disabilities* (pp. 3–33). New York, NY: Springer-Verlag.

Larson, V.L., & McKinley, N. (1987). *Communication assessment and intervention strategies for adolescents.* Eau Claire, WI: Thinking Publications.

Lytle, S.L., & Cochran-Smith, M. (1992). Teacher research as a way of knowing. *Harvard Educational Review, 62,* 447–474.

McTear, M.F., & Conti-Ramsden, G. (1992). *Pragmatic disability in children.* San Diego, CA: Singular.

Paulson, F., Paulson, P., & Meyer, C. (1991). What makes a portfolio a portfolio? *Educational Leadership, 48,* 60–63.

Rees, N.S., & Gerber, S. (1992). Ethnography and communication: Social-role relations. *Topics in Language Disorders, 12* (3), 15–27.

Scott, C.M. (1989). Problem writers: Nature, assessment, and intervention. In A.G. Kamhi & H.W. Catts (Eds.), *Reading disabilities: A developmental language perspective* (pp. 303–344). Boston, MA: College-Hill.

Silliman, E.R., & Wilkinson, L.C. (1991). *Communicating for learning: Classroom observation and collaboration.* Gaithersburg, MD: Aspen.

Silliman, E.R., & Wilkinson, L.C. (in press-a). Discourse scaffolds for classroom intervention. In G.P. Wallach & K.G. Butler (Eds.), *Language learning disabilities in school-age children and adolescents* (2nd ed.). Columbus, OH: Merrill.

Silliman, E.R., & Wilkinson, L.C. (in press-b). Observation

is more than looking. Assessing students' progress in classroom language learning. In G.P. Wallach & K.G. Butler (Eds.), *Language learning disabilities in school-age children and adolescents* (2nd ed.). Columbus, OH: Merrill.

Westby, C.E., & Costlow, L. (1991). Implementing a whole language program in a special education class. *Topics in Language Disorders, 11* (3), 69–84.

Wilkinson, L.C., & Silliman, E.R. (in press). Assessing progress in language and literacy: A classroom approach. In L.M. Morrow, J. Smith, & L.C. Wilkinson (Eds.), *The integrated language arts: Controversy to consensus.* Newton, MA: Allyn & Bacon.

Comprehension of meaning in written language

Nancy A. Creaghead, PhD
Associate Professor
Communication Department
University of Cincinnati
Cincinnati, Ohio

DOES THE communication specialist—the person whose expertise has traditionally been in oral language—have a role in the teaching of reading? If so, what can the communication specialist contribute to helping children comprehend meaning in written language?

Some compelling arguments exist for including the oral language specialist on the "reading team." Perhaps the most important factor to consider is the close relationship between oral and written language skills. Henderson (1969) states, "The Piaget model suggests that beginning-to-read is an integral part of an overall language development" (p. 91). Furthermore, the language experience model of teaching reading (Gans, 1979; Hall, 1970; Stouffer, 1970) is based on the premise that children's oral language production is closely related to, and an important source of instructional stimuli for, beginning reading. That related language skills underlie both oral and written communication is further supported by the fact that

TLD, 1986, 6(4), 73–82
© 1986 Aspen Publishers, Inc.

children with oral language disorders are at risk for reading problems (Creaghead & Donnelly, 1982; Hasenstab & Laughton, 1982).

Given the premise of the unity of oral and written language, it follows that the language specialist has certain expertise that applies to reading. As a form of language, written communication is composed of the familiar components: pragmatics, semantics, syntax, morphology, and a graphological system, which is parallel to the phonological system in oral language. In what Goodman (1967) calls a "psycholinguistic guessing game," readers extract meaning from written language by sampling, predicting, testing, and confirming hypotheses about content. They do this based on knowledge of the overall format and structure of text (pragmatics), meaning (semantics and derivational morphology), sentence structure (syntax and inflectional morphology), and phoneme-grapheme correspondences (graphology-phonology). In other words, comprehending written language involves processes that correspond directly to those that are necessary for comprehending oral language.

In viewing the relationship between written language comprehension and oral language comprehension, it is possible to identify some ways in which the language specialist can support language-delayed children *and* the reading teacher by applying language-learning principles.

COMPREHENSION AND PRODUCTION IN READING AND WRITING

One such principle is that normal children learn to comprehend and produce language at nearly the same time. In fact, researchers have found it difficult to separate some facets of comprehension and production in early language development (Bloom & Lahey, 1978). Likewise, Durkin (1966) found that interest in writing was a common characteristic of children who learned to read early, and it has been observed that providing experience in writing encourages better reading skills (Dobson, 1985; Hall, 1970; Strickland, 1969). Thus the following discussion will consider the child both as a reader and as a writer. This approach is based on the idea that development of the two skills is interrelated in the same way that comprehension and production are interrelated in oral language development, and that development of certain writing skills may even enhance reading comprehension.

THE ROLE OF FUNCTION IN MEANING

One important semantic/pragmatic fact is that language that is functional for the young child is meaningful to him or her. Children communicate to fulfill a purpose. Halliday (1977, p. 37) observed the following functions in the communicative repertoire of his 22-month-old child: (a) instrumental—requesting objects; (b) regulatory—directing actions; (c) interactional—relating socially; (d) personal—showing off and expressing feelings; (e) heuristic—requesting information; (f) imaginative—making believe; and (g) informative—providing information.

Written language also serves a variety of purposes. For example, adults use written language to request refunds (instrumental), to request services (regulatory), to keep in touch (interactional), to create poetry (personal), to solicit advice (heuristic), to write novels (imaginative), and to give directions (informative). In addition, Lindfors (1980) notes that school-age children use oral language for an even wider range of functions than preschoolers, and that these also correspond to written language purposes.

In contrast, what is the apparent function of the written language that is often presented to beginning readers? In such materials, the overriding, and often exclusive, purpose is to teach the child to read. Normal children do not listen in order to learn language, nor do they talk in order to learn to talk. They listen in order to extract meaning from messages, and they talk in order to fulfill some communicative purpose. When children read aloud in class they are learning to call words more than they are learning to extract meaning. To the extent that written language fulfills some communicative purpose for children, their interest, comprehension, and spontaneous use are increasingly probable.

The language specialist can enhance the development of functional written communication by incorporating useful written messages into language instruction. As part of a language experience, the clinician can provide written directions for completing an activity. One child, in turn, can write directions for others to read and follow. Both writing directions and following them require organization and sequencing skills that are important for school activities such as completing workbook pages and written tests. Other functional activities involving reading might include a treasure hunt, using a shopping list, or reading brochures to decide where to go on a field trip. The important point is that, in each case, the child must extract meaning in order to fulfill some goal.

In making the transition from functional to academic reading, the stories from classroom "readers" can be made more meaningful by using them as a basis for picture drawing, discussion of characters or problems raised in the stories, role playing, writing plays, and other oral and written activities. Again, emphasis should be placed on extracting meaning rather than on calling words.

Author and audience considerations for making meaning clear

Delineating the function of a communicative act presupposes a specific sender and receiver. These roles are referred to as *author* and *audience* in written language communication. Problems arise if the purpose of written communication is unclear to the child. The author and the audience may be ambiguous to the child also. In oral language learning, children know to whom they are directing communication, and those who communicate with them frame their messages with the child's needs in mind. That is, children learn to communicate in an environment in which speakers give careful attention to ensuring that children comprehend messages (Snow, 1977).

For example, in communicating orally with young children, adults consider not only the children's linguistic abilities, but also what they know about the topic and the degree to which the context can support their comprehension. Snow (1977) notes that in communicating with young children, adults provide support for learning about conversations by carrying the burden of the communicative interaction and allowing the child to participate at his or her level. Greater expectations for responses occur gradually as the child's comprehension of questions and communication skills increases.

In such an environment, children learn to appreciate the needs of the listener, and they learn to expect that messages should be comprehensible. In oral communication situations, the audience is clear, and it is an important factor in determining the nature of the message. For example, children often produce inadequate messages, in which necessary new information is omitted. A child may say, "It's brown." In this situation, an adult will request clarification, "What's brown?" giving the child information about how to meet the needs of the listener when the child is the speaker, and providing a model for requesting clarification when the child is the listener.

Written language requires more *verbal* context and information because of the reduced *visual* and *situational* context available to the reader, accompanied by the reader's inability to request clarification from the author. Personalized written communication can bridge the gap between personal oral communication

Personalized written communication can bridge the gap between personal oral communication and the kind of depersonalization that exists in written language intended for larger audiences.

and the kind of depersonalization that exists in written language intended for larger audiences. Reading from basal readers may not give children the idea that written messages have meaning for them; but a note from the teacher may help them to see themselves as the intended audience. Incorporating not only purpose, but also a clear idea of the writer and reader into early written language activities promotes reading comprehension because the child can view the written message as a communicative event that includes an expectation of personalized meaning for him or her.

The use of experience stories in teaching written language comprehension has the advantage of including the child both as author and audience. In preparing such stories, the language specialist can match written material to the child's language and reading level by eliciting ideas from the child and then writing them on paper, initially to be read for or with the child. Ideas expressed by children can be expanded in regard to both meaning and form so that the children can read material that is within the realm of their experience but increases their ability to use linguistic skills for reading.

When adults use written messages to communicate to specific children (e.g., giving directions, sharing ideas, asking questions, creating a poem about a shared experience), these children see themselves as the intended audience. Likewise, when children write for a specific audience with a clear purpose, they learn to give attention to the needs of that audience.

The communication specialist is in a position to help children understand how author and audience concerns are important in making written language meaningful through individual discussion of written communication. This might be accomplished by discussing written material such as problem-solving tasks or through practical applications of written messages, as in directions or games (e.g., "Why didn't you know what to do? What else should the author have told you?"). The transition to more formal reading material can be made through metalinguistic discussion of authors and their purposes, or by generating clarification questions that readers might ask authors if they were available.

Reference considerations for making meaning clear

Research indicates that children under age 7 have difficulty taking the perspective of the listener in order to make their meaning clear for the listener in an oral barrier game task (Brown, 1983; Glucksberg, Krauss, & Higgins, 1975; Whitehurst & Sonnenschein, 1981). This task involves communicating about a referent to a listener who does not share a visual context with the speaker to have the listener select or act on a particular object in a particular way. As speakers, children at this age are unable to provide completely informative messages that specify the referent verbally.

Research has examined whether this difficulty is a result of egocentric behavior, in that the child ignores the listener's needs, or of an inability to identify the critical elements to be communicated. It appears that both factors may be involved (Asher & Wigfield, 1981; Glucksberg, Krauss, & Higgins, 1975; Whitehurst &

Sonnenschein, 1981). In addition, it has been found that, when observing communication failure between two other people, children blame the listener or receiver rather than determining that a message did not provide the critical information (Robinson & Robinson, 1976). The converse of the expressive difficulty is also observed, in that children as listeners have difficulty identifying the inadequacy of messages. However, referential skills do appear to improve during the school-age years, until grade five, when children are able to perform like adults on many barrier tasks (Buerkle, 1983).

The barrier game task shares elements with written language in the sense that visual context is eliminated, and comprehension is dependent on verbal communication alone. If children are unable to evaluate the informativeness of messages, they will be unable to determine the reason for their own comprehension failures and will have difficulty asking the questions necessary to be successful at the "psycholinguistic guessing game" of reading (Goodman, 1967). Language-delayed children exhibit this problem in regard to oral communication. They may operate on the implicit assumption that verbal messages do not make sense, and therefore may not learn how and when to ask appropriate clarification questions. These children, and other children with reading comprehension problems, often exhibit the same behavior in reading.

When teachers provide support for children's early written communication attempts in order to ensure that messages make sense, children's referential skills are likely to improve, and reading and writing ability may be enhanced. For example, if the language specialist writes a message to a child, the child has the opportunity to request clarification in order to understand, and the adult can interact with the child to support comprehension. Barrier games can be used to enhance both oral and written comprehension of messages and bridge the gap to information that is not supported by immediate shared context. A series of activities sequenced in order of difficulty might include the following:

- The adult provides oral directions to the child across a barrier, and encourages the child to ask clarification questions to complete the task.
- The adult tape-records directions for the child to follow, and the child must follow the directions without asking questions, although he or she might formulate questions or suggest improved directions in subsequent discussion.
- The adult provides written directions for the child to follow in completing a task.

At this written language level, the child could formulate questions or improved directions either orally or in writing. In this activity, as in others, the task of formulating effective messages can be helpful in increasing comprehension of them.

The importance of scripts and formats in deriving meaning

Children learn language in meaningful contexts. Development of comprehension is aided by contextual clues, which include the event structure, the child's script knowledge, and a variety of nonverbal clues. A number of authors (Creaghead & Tattershall, 1985; Lund & Duchan, 1983; Rumelhart, 1984) have discussed the role

of scripts and schemas in language learning and comprehension. As children develop a script for an event, they are able to encode appropriate language to fit that event script. Examples of such scripts are going to a restaurant, participating in preschool snacktime or sharing time, taking a test, or playing kickball on the playground.

Script development can occur for every imaginable repeatable activity through multiple similar experiences with the activity. An adequate script is not usually developed through one or two experiences of the event, but through multiple ones. In the context of the multiple experiences, children learn to detect the factors that remain constant, and thus define the script, versus those that may vary within certain limits, which again are defined by the script. Imagine the example of an adult who has been to one airport. No matter how many times the individual has visited this airport, the experience will not provide an adequate script for predicting airport formats. There is no reason to predict that all airports will be like this one. Visits to a number of airports, however, will enable the development of a script that will help the traveler predict how to get through any airport.

Similarly, children must learn how to predict meaning in written language by using their knowledge of scripts and text formats. Written language has a text structure that can aid comprehension. Researchers (Bransford & Johnson, 1972; Calfee & Curley, 1984; Mandler & Johnson, 1977; Thorndyke, 1977) have examined the influence of text structure on comprehension and have found that adults show better comprehension of information that is organized cohesively.

Creaghead and Tattershall (1985) have also demonstrated the importance of *format* in children's comprehension of written directions like those found in workbooks. Characteristics of text format, such as the title and subheadings (Hasenstab & Laughton, 1982), pictures (Porter, 1969), page layout (Creaghead & Tattershall, 1985), and overall organization (Page & Stewart, 1985), give clues as to the purpose of the text and the type of information to be found.

For example, a personal letter has a visual format that clues the reader to certain potential communicative characteristics, such as that the information may be directed to the reader personally and not to a wider audience. The return address alerts the reader to other clues about the nature of the information within the body of the letter. On the other hand, initial reading material is often presented in only one format (the preprimer), and that format may be distorted with the idea of making it simpler. For example, sentences may be presented on separate lines, like a poem, rather than in paragraph form. Reading comprehension may be fostered by providing materials whose overall format aids in detection of a clear purpose. Children also may need direct instruction regarding how to make use of varied formats to predict content.

One oral language format, which is based on scripts, and is common in the early reading material presented to children, is narration. Children who are read to at home experience the narrative style and have the opportunity to develop knowledge of the predictable structure of "story grammar," which they can later use in comprehending other stories they hear or read (Mandler & Johnson, 1977; Stein,

1979). Language-delayed children often have difficulty or limited experience with this structure (Graybeal, 1981). Parents of young language-delayed children may report that their children do not like to be read to or to listen to stories. The language specialist can intervene in this maladaptive cycle, and can assist children to develop a sense of narration and story grammar by providing oral experiences that match the child's linguistic and experience levels, and by gradually relating these experiences to written texts read aloud.

Using context to predict meaning

Children comprehend the meaning of what is said to them partly by making predictions based on the context in which the language is presented. This context includes the purpose or function of the communication, the speaker and listener, the referent, and the script. Although all of these variables are important, they are not the only sources of meaning. To comprehend the sentence, "The cat's claws are sharp, and if he scratches you, you will get a laceration," the child does not have to have known the meaning of the word, "laceration" previously. He or she can extract it from the verbal or semantic context. If the child has had prior experience with cat scratches, he or she will have an even clearer picture of this particular type of laceration. This is the typical way in which children learn the meaning of new words.

Smith (1978) has described a similar process in the development of reading comprehension. Good readers predict meaning on the basis of the prior experience that they bring to the text (e.g., experience with cats); on the basis of the meaning of the other words in the sentence (e.g., *scratch–laceration*); and on the basis of the syntax (e.g., *laceration* must be a noun). Poor readers may not try to predict meaning, or they may have deficient prediction strategies. Some poor readers may not be able to determine which part of a complex message is important for answering a given question (Creaghead & Donnelly, 1982). Teaching children to expect meaning and to use effective prediction strategies can improve reading comprehension.

Because language-delayed children may not have developed the linguistic skills needed for effective prediction of complex reading material, the language specialist may play a dual role. On the one hand, it may be necessary to rewrite some academic materials in order to make the prediction task easier. Providing redundancy and clear meaning links for new words in written material are two ways to give children success in prediction. On the other hand, it is important to give children the tools and strategies for comprehending new meanings by providing experiences (and accompanying vocabulary) related to the material to be read. Children may also need direct instruction in how to use prior experience, pictures, format, linguistic context, and other predictors to extract meaning.

AN INTEGRATED EXPERIENCE APPROACH TO READING

Language experiences have been suggested as a strategy for initiating reading comprehension (Gans, 1979; Hall, 1970; Henderson, 1969; Stouffer, 1970). In later elementary grades, children are expected to use their acquired reading skills to get information from textbooks and other reference materials. Increasing demands for comprehension are imposed as materials include more sophisticated ideas and concepts, increased use of figurative language, new vocabulary, and more complex text structure and sentences. Although many children make the adjustment easily, some children need continued support to meet the demands. These children may need to be taught strategies for using titles, subheadings, and text structure to get the main idea; for using context to understand new vocabulary and figurative expressions; and for understanding the perspective of the writer and the reader in order to evaluate opinions.

Older children with limited reading skills also need continued exposure to varied reading experiences, accompanied by increased focus on the different strategies required for each type of experience. However, it often happens that they receive less variety of reading opportunity than the more capable students. While slower students labor over textbooks, gifted students may participate in projects that provide opportunities to expand their range of reading experiences and styles of writing. Examples include producing television shows and plays, planning field trips, and getting involved in current events. It is just these kinds of activities,

---

While slower students labor over textbooks, gifted students may participate in projects that provide opportunities to expand their range of reading experiences and styles of writing.

---

with their practical and communicative focus, that may aid poorer readers in increasing their skills and interest.

A newspaper is one example of a way in which comprehension and production of oral and written language can be integrated into a functional communication task for older children. The characteristics of the activity are as follows:

1. On the basis of Halliday's (1977) taxonomy, the following communicative functions may be included in a newspaper: news reports, advice column, entertainment reviews (informative), letters to advice column (heuristic), cartoons, poetry, stories (imaginative or personal), editorials, and advertisements (regulatory).

2. Reading for purposive comprehension can be incorporated. Demands for thoughtful reading include reading other newspapers to get ideas, reading news and reference sources for background information, reading books in order to write reviews, and proofreading. The comprehension strategies and demands for each of these activities is different, and each relates to reading activities needed in school. For example, in looking for ideas, the student may read for generalities; reference sources may be used to extract details; reviewing requires consideration of style and interest; proofreading demands attention to mechanics.

3. The purpose and the audience for written material can be made clear. When the newspaper is actually distributed to a predetermined audience, the concept of old and new information can be discussed in relationship to what must be made clear in the article so that readers will understand.

4. Oral language activities can be integrated with written activities. In order to report events, children must be provided with notable experiences. To give background information, they must take polls, interview participants, and ask questions. In order to review books, plays, and musical events, they must read or view them and then discuss them to form opinions.

5. The format for various types of writing can be made clear and distinct. The newspaper provides a perfect example of information that is designed so that the reader is able to use the format to organize his reading and to get information quickly and easily. A table of contents tells where information is located. Headlines provide a statement of the topic. Major sections and regular features are marked by recognizable visual features, and the writing in each section has its own unique style.

• • •

An integrated experience project helps children learn to comprehend written language by putting meaning in the forefront and providing the opportunity for children to learn strategies for comprehending and producing a variety of types of material. Many other projects can be used to the same advantage. The language specialist is in a unique position to use such activities to assist language-impaired children to use meaning in the comprehension and production of oral and written language.

REFERENCES

Asher, S.R., & Wigfield, A. (1981). Training referential communication skills. In W.P. Dickson (Ed.), *Children's oral communication skills*. New York: Academic Press.

Bloom L., & Lahey, M. (1978). Language development and language disorders. New York: John Wiley and Sons.

Bransford, J.D., & Johnson, M.K. (1972). Contextual prerequisites for understanding: Some investigations of comprehension and recall. *Journal of Verbal Learning and Verbal Behavior, 11,* 717–726

Brown, J. (1983) *Communication skills of normal first grade children involved in a direction giving task using a barrier game*. Unpublished master's thesis, University of Cinicnnati.

Buerkle, J. (1983). A *study of communication and revision strategies used by fifth graders involved in a direction giving task within the context of a communication barrier game*. Unpublished master's thesis, University of Cincinnati.

Calfee, R.C., & Curley, R. (1984). Structures of prose in the content areas. In J. Flood (Ed.), *Understanding reading comprehension: Cognition, language and the structure of prose*. Newark, DE: International Reading Association.

Creaghead, N.A., & Donnelly, K.G. (1982). Comprehension of superordinate and subordinate information by good and poor readers. *Language, Speech and Hearing Services in the Schools, 13,* 177–186.

Creaghead, N.A., & Tattershall, S.S. (1985). Observation and assessment of classroom pragmatic skills. In C. Simon (Ed.), *Communication skills and classroom success*. San Diego, CA: College-Hill Press.

Dobson, L.N. (1985). Learn to read by writing: A practical program for reluctant readers. *Teaching Exceptional Children, 18,* Fall, 30–36.

Durkin, D. (1966). *Children who read early*. New York: Teachers College Press.

Gans, R. (1979). *Guiding children's reading through experiences*. New York: Teachers College Press.

Glucksberg, S., Krauss, R., & Higgins, E. (1975). The development of referential communication skills. In F. Horowitz (Ed.), *Review of child development research* (Vol. 4). Chicago: University of Chicago Press.

Goodman, K.S. (1967). Reading: A psycholinguistic guessing game. *Journal of the Reading Specialist, 6,* 126–135.

Graybeal, C.M. (1981). Memory for stories in language-impaired children. *Applied Psycholinguistics, 2,* 269–283.

Hall, M. (1970). *Teaching reading as a language experience*. Columbus, OH: Charles E. Merrill.

Halliday, M.A.K. (1977). *Learning how to mean*. New York: Elsevier North Holland.

Hasenstab, M.S., & Laughton, J. (1982). *Reading, writing, and the exceptional child: A psycho-socio-linguistic approach*. Rockville, MD: Aspen Systems.

Henderson, E.H. (1969). Do we apply what we know about comprehension? In N.H. Smith (Ed.), *Current issues in reading*. Newark, DE: International Reading Association.

Lindfors, J. (1980). *Children's language and learning*. Englewood Cliffs, NJ: Prentice-Hall.

Lund, N., & Duchan, J. (1983). *Assessing children's language in naturalistic contexts*. Englewood Cliffs, NJ: Prentice-Hall.

Mandler, J.M., & Johnson, N.S. (1977). Remembrance of things parsed: Story structure and recall. *Cognitive Psychology, 9,* 111–151.

Page, J., & Stewart, S. (1985). Story grammar skills in school-age children. *Topics in Language Disorders, 5,* 16–30.

Porter, P. (1969). Pictures in reading. *The Reading Teacher, 22,* 238–241.

Robinson, E.J., & Robinson, W.P. (1976). Developmental changes in the child's explanation of communication failure. *Australian Journal of Psychology, 29,* 101–109.

Rumelhart, D.E. (1984). Understanding understanding. In J. Flood (Ed.), *Understanding reading comprehension: Cognition, language and the structure of prose*. Newark, DE: International Reading Association.

Smith, F. (1978). *Reading without nonsense*. New York: Teachers College Press.

Snow, C.E. (1977). The development of conversation between mothers and babies. *Journal of Child Language, 4,* 1–22.

Stein, N.L. (1979). How children understand stories: A developmental analysis. In L. Katz (Ed.), *Current topics in early childhood education* (Vol. 2). Norwood, NJ: Ablex.

Stouffer, R. (1970). *The language experience approach to the teaching of reading*. New York: Harper and Row.

Strickland, R.G. (1969). Building on what we know. In J.A. Figurel (Ed.), *Reading and realism*. Newark, DE: International Reading Association.

Thorndyke, P.W. (1977). Cognitive structures in comprehension and memory of narrative discourse. *Cognitive Psychology, 9,* 77–110.

Whitehurst, G.J., & Sonnenschein, S. (1981). The development of informative messages in referential communication: Knowing when versus knowing how. In W.P. Dickson (Ed.), *Children's oral communication skills*. New York: Academic Press.

Early identification of reading disabilities

Hugh W. Catts, PhD
Department of Speech-Language-Hearing:
  Sciences and Disorders
University of Kansas
Lawrence, Kansas

EACH YEAR, thousands of children experience significant difficulties in learning to read and are diagnosed as having a specific learning or reading disability. Typically, this diagnosis is made during the primary grades and is based on a child's poor performance on tests of reading achievement in the face of adequate scores on measures of intellectual and sensory abilities. For many reading-disabled children, however, this diagnosis comes only after considerable academic failure. Because these children are often not identified until they are 9 or 10 years of age, many of them have struggled with learning to read for several years. This struggle often leads to poor motivation and negative attitudes toward reading as well as more serious socioemotional problems (Johnston & Winograd, 1985). In an attempt to limit reading. failure and the negative consequences of this failure, researchers and practitioners have focused on the early identification of reading dis-

Top Lang Disord, 1991,12(1),1–16
© 1991 Aspen Publishers, Inc.

abilities (e.g., Jansky & De Hirsch, 1972; Masland & Masland, 1988).

A major obstacle for early identification is the lack of an adequate conceptualization or definition of a specific reading disability.* Traditionally, a specific reading disability has been defined as difficulty in learning to read in the absence of low intelligence, sensory deficits, or the lack of opportunity (Critchely, 1970). Like traditional definitions, most definitions used today are exclusionary in nature. That is, they define the problem by excluding factors known to be associated with learning problems in general. As such, they tell us much more about what the disorder is not rather than what it is. In most definitions, the only explicitly stated symptom of the disorder is the presence of reading difficulties. Therefore, when employing these definitions, we are forced to await the appearance of reading problems before identifying the disability.

Clearly, what is necessary to improve early identification is a more comprehensive conceptualization of the disorder, one that provides an account of the characteristics associated with a reading disability throughout development, especially in the preschool years. Fortunately, over the last 10 to 15 years, significant advancements have been made in the field of reading disabilities, and these advancements have now begun to lead to an understanding of the developmental course of reading disabilities. Specifically, a number of investigators have proposed that in many cases a reading disability is a reflection of a developmental language disorder (Catts, 1989a; Chasty, 1985; Kamhi & Catts, 1989; Liberman & Shankweiler, 1985; Scarborough, 1990; Vellutino, 1979). It is argued that

this disorder begins early in life and continues throughout childhood, adolescence, and into adulthood. The manifestation of the language disorder, however, changes with development. A large body of research now demonstrates that in many cases the early manifestations of a reading disability are difficulties in oral language (see Kamhi & Catts, 1989; Wagner & Torgesen, 1987). Research further shows that these difficulties usually continue into the school years and occur alongside problems in learning to read, write, and spell (Bishop & Adams, 1990; Kamhi & Catts, 1986; Tallal, Curtiss, & Kaplan, 1989; Wolf & Obregon, 1989). In this article, research concerning the language basis of reading disabilities will be examined, and implications will be considered for the early identification of reading disabilities.

LANGUAGE PROBLEMS IN READING-DISABLED CHILDREN

The language basis of reading disabilities has been examined from several different perspectives. One body of research has focused on the oral language problems observed in children with reading disabilities (for review, see Aaron, 1989; Roth & Spekman, 1989a). Generally, this has involved selecting a group of school-age children identified as reading disabled (or in some cases as learning disabled) and examining their performance on traditional speech and language measures. This work has demonstrated that reading-disabled (RD) children often have problems in the use and/or comprehension of morphology and syntax (Doehring, Trites, Patel, & Fiederowicz, 1981; Fletcher, Satz, & Scholes, 1981; Vogel, 1974). Language deficits have also been reported in the production of narratives (Feagans & Short, 1984; Roth & Spekman, 1989b), comprehension of figurative language (Seindenberg & Berstein, 1986), and the use of text-level comprehension strategies (Donahue, 1984; Short & Ryan, 1984).

Although this research has indicated that RD children have various deficits in oral language, it is unclear what this work tells us about the language basis of reading disabilities. A major problem for the interpretation of this research is that language abilities and reading performance/deficits have been examined concurrently. That is, children were already displaying reading disabilities when their language skills were examined. As such, it is unclear whether language problems represent antecedent conditions (i.e., early manifestations) or, conversely, the consequences of a reading disability. The latter is certainly a viable alternative. Reading, being a linguistic activity, exposes children to language and thus provides an excellent opportunity for language learning. In fact, during the school years, children may be exposed to more abstract vocabulary and complex language structure in print than in spoken language. Because of their reading problems, RD children do not have the same opportunity to learn language from reading and therefore may show language deficits when compared to their normal reading peers (Donahue, 1986; Stanovich, 1986).

Not all studies of the language problems of RD children have investigated language and reading problems concurrently. Several investigations have examined language development in children before their school entrance and their identification as reading disabled. For example, in a retrospective study, Ingram, Mason, and Blackburn (1970) investigated the early language development of 62 children with specific reading disabilities. Detailed developmental histories of these subjects indicated that 56% displayed preschool speech and language difficulties.

An especially well-designed study of the early language development of RD children was recently completed by Scarborough (1990, 1991). In this investigation, a group of 2½-year-old children ($N = 34$) with a family history of a significant childhood reading disability (parent or older sibling) and a control group ($N = 44$) with no such family history were selected and followed periodically through the second grade. Of the 34 children with a family history of reading difficulties, 22 subsequently were found to have a significant reading disability in the second grade (referred to as the dyslexic subjects). Scarborough compared performance on a limited set of language measures by the dyslexic subjects at 30, 36, 42, 48, and 60 months to that of a matched subgroup of control subjects. Results indicated that the dyslexic subjects performed significantly more poorly than the normal subjects on a measure of receptive language processing (Northwestern Syntax Screening Test [NSST]) at 36 and 48 months but not at 60 months (NSST was not given at 30 and 42 months). Dyslexic subjects were also found to produce syntactically less complex sentences and had a shorter mean length of utterance (MLU) than control subjects at 30, 36, 42, and 48 months but, again, not at 60 months. An examination of individual subject data revealed that early difficulties in expressive syntax were fairly consistent across the dyslexic subjects. This was supported by a discriminant analysis that indicated that early syntactic proficiency predicted group membership (i.e., dyslexic or normal) with 77% accuracy.

Although syntactic difficulties did discriminate between reading groups, the severity of these difficulties was not closely related to later reading achievement in the dyslexic group. That is, dyslexic subjects with the lowest reading scores in the second grade were not necessarily those with the most delayed syntax in the preschool years. It also should be noted that, whereas statistically significant group differences were observed in expressive syntax at 30 months, these differences do not necessarily indicate that the dyslexic children had a clinically significant problem, at least not according to traditional criteria. The dyslexic group's mean MLU at 30 months was well within the normal range specified by Miller and Chapman (1981). More importantly, none of the dyslexic subjects were identified for speech-language services during the preschool years (H. Scarborough, personal communication). This does not, however, diminish the significance of the dyslexics' problems in expressive syntax. Rather, it suggests that these problems may be less severe or more subtle than those discussed below for specific language-impaired (LI) children.

Finally, Scarborough's finding that 65% of the children with a family history of reading disabilities later demonstrated reading problems themselves is a strong indication of the familial nature of the disorder (also see Pennington, 1989). A positive family history of a reading disability may be an early sign of a potential reading problem, particularly when accompanied by preschool language difficulties.

FOLLOW-UP STUDIES OF LANGUAGE-IMPAIRED CHILDREN

Another line of inquiry that is contributing to the understanding of the language basis of reading disabilities is the longitudinal investigation of specific LI children. In this work, children displaying significant language impairments (i.e., language abilities 1 to 2 standard deviations [SDs] below the mean) have been identified in preschool or kindergarten and tested for reading and academic achievement in the primary grades (Aram & Nation, 1980; Bishop & Adams, 1990; Hall & Tomblin, 1978; Silva, McGee, & Williams, 1987; Stark et al., 1984; Tallal et al., 1989; Wilson & Risucci, 1988; also see for review Aram & Hall, 1989; Weiner, 1985). The results of this body of research have consistently shown that LI children are at risk for reading and learning disabilities. The percentage of LI children found later to display reading disabilities, however, does vary considerably across investigations. Some researchers have reported that as little as 25% of LI children have subsequent reading disabilities (e.g., Bishop & Adams, 1990), whereas others have found that well over half these children have reading problems (Stark et al., 1984; Tallal et al., 1989). The inconsistency in these findings is, in part, the result of differences

---

A positive family history of a reading disability may be an early sign of a potential reading problem, particularly when accompanied by preschool language difficulties.

---

in the way reading disabilities are measured. Studies vary greatly in choice of reading achievement measures (i.e., word recognition vs. reading comprehension tests) and cut-off values for determining a significant reading problem (e.g., 1 SD vs. 2 SD below the mean).

The variability in the reported academic outcome of LI children also may be due to sampling differences among the studies. LI children are known to represent a heterogeneous group, and individual differences in cognitive-linguistic abilities among subjects within and across studies could account, in part, for differences in reading achievement. For example, it has been proposed that reading outcome may be related to the degree of specificity of the language impairment, that is, whether the impairment is specific to language deficits or part of a more general cognitive dysfunction (Bishop & Adams, 1990). As with most studies of LI children, longitudinal investigations have typically sought to exclude children with general developmental delays. Among the LI subjects in some longitudinal studies, however, there have been a number of children who have displayed low nonverbal cognitive abilities in addition to language deficits. In a recent investigation, Bishop and Adams (1990) conducted a follow-up study of 82 children identified as being language impaired at 4 years of age. Although sampling procedures were designed to exclude children with general intellectual retardation, a subgroup of children ($N = 19$) was found to demonstrate poor nonverbal abilities when tested by the investigators (i.e., >2 SD below the control group mean on a modified version of the Leiter International Performance Scale;

see Bishop & Edmundson, 1987). When examined 4 years later, this subgroup of children was found to be more than twice as likely to have a reading disability as subjects who initially had verbal deficits alone.

Whereas Bishop and Adams' (1990) results indicate that LI children with poor nonverbal abilities are at a high risk for reading failure, other studies of LI children have not found a strong relationship between reading and nonverbal abilities when the latter abilities have been within the normal range (e.g., ± 2 SDs of the mean; e.g., Catts, 1991; Tallal et al., 1989). In addition, investigations of reading development in much wider cross-sections of children (not limited to LI children) have failed to find a strong association between nonverbal abilities and reading achievement (see Hessler, 1987; Stanovich, 1991). This research has indicated that it is verbal abilities, not nonverbal abilities, that are most closely related to reading development.

Beyond general cognitive factors, research suggests that the type or level of language impairment is an important variable in predicting academic/reading outcome. Specifically, research has demonstrated that deficits in the semantic-syntactic aspects of language are associated more often with reading disabilities than difficulties that are restricted to phonology (at least in the way in which the latter difficulties have traditionally been defined; but see the discussion below concerning phonological processing deficits). For example, Levi, Capozzi, Fabrizi, and Sechi (1982) identified two groups of 3- to 4-year-old children: one group with predominately phonological impairments

(PI group) and the other with deficits both at the phonological and semantic-syntactic levels (LI group). At the end of first grade, the LI group performed less well than the PI group on tests of reading achievement. Specifically, a third of the LI group showed poor reading achievement, half showed mediocre performance, and only two subjects displayed good achievement. In contrast, among the members of the PI group, only one subject demonstrated poor reading achievement, half the subjects showed mediocre performance, and about half showed good achievement.

Bishop and Adams (1990) have also reported that young children with phonological disorders alone are less likely to have subsequent reading problems than those with other types of language deficits. In fact, they found that the former group of children were not at all at risk for reading disabilities. Among their 82 LI subjects, 12 displayed primarily phonological disorders at 4½ years of age. Phonological disorders, measured by percentage of consonant correct on a picture-naming task, were mild in 1 case, mild to moderate in 7, and severe in 4. This subgroup of subjects was found to demonstrate above average reading abilities when tested at 8½ years of age. Bishop and Adams (1990) further found that, when all 82 subjects were considered, phonological ability at 4½ years of age did not correlate significantly with later reading achievement. When phonological ability was examined at 5½ years of age, however, it was found to correlate with later reading but accounted for only a small percentage of the variance (also see Hall & Tomblin, 1978; Shriberg & Kwiatkowski, 1988).

Whereas Bishop and Adams (1990) found

that children with early phonological disorders alone were not at risk for later reading disabilities, they reported that preschool children with semantic-syntactic impairments often did develop reading problems. Bishop and Adams (and Bishop & Edmundson, 1987) tested the language abilities of their LI children at 4½ and 5½ years of age and then measured their reading achievement at age 8½. Their results revealed that a subgroup of LI subjects identified at 4½ years of age had improved significantly in language skills and were nearly normal at age 5½. Among these 29 subjects (details were not provided, and as many as 12 of these subjects may have had problems limited to phonology), only 1 child later displayed a reading disability. On the other hand, children who continued to show language impairments at 5½ years of age were found to be at a much greater risk of having a reading disability. It was observed that 25% of the latter children displayed reading difficulties at 8½ years of age. This percentage is much lower than that reported in most studies, but a reading disability was defined by a more stringent criterion than that used in many other studies involving LI children (i.e., reading performance more than 1.96 SDs below that predicted by nonverbal IQ). Finally, of particular note, Bishop and Adams (1990) found that among the language measures given at 4½ and 5½ years of age, MLU was the best predictor of reading and spelling abilities at age 8½.

In another recent longitudinal study, Tallal et al. (1989) identified 67 LI and 54 matched normal children at 4 years of age and evaluated them annually through 8 years of age on perceptual-motor, language, cognitive, prereading, and academic skills. They reported that, upon entering school, the LI children performed significantly less well in reading than the normal control group. Group differences in reading ability were further found to increase over time and by age 8 approximately 66% of the LI children were reading at a level that was at least 1 SD below the mean for the normal control subjects. Regression analyses indicated that preschool measures of perceptual-motor skills (e.g., nonverbal sequencing, repeating *pa/ta/ka* in rapid succession) were the best predictors of reading achievement in the LI children. Severity of preschool language impairment was not significantly related to later reading achievement. Preschool language abilities, however, particularly receptive skills, were found to be a good predictor of school placement for the most academically delayed children. That is, the LI children who continued to have academic problems in the primary grades and who were in special education classes at age 8 most often had receptive language deficits at age 4.

Wilson and Risucci (1988) also have reported that preschool receptive language disorders may be predictive of later academic difficulties. They investigated 72 LI children 3 to 4 years of age who were attending an early intervention program. Subjects were divided into four groups on the basis of their language deficits. These included children with problems in (1) receptive language, (2) auditory memory and word retrieval, (3) expressive formulation, and (4) organizational aspects of language. When reading achievement was examined in grades 1 to 4, it was observed that subjects with preschool receptive lan-

guage problems or auditory memory and word retrieval deficits had a 30% to 50% chance of demonstrating a reading disability. Children with preschool expressive and/or organizational deficits were observed to be much less at risk for reading failure (0% to 30%).

Most recently, Catts (1991) examined 41 kindergarten children with speech-language impairments. Standardized testing by the investigators indicated that 28 of these children displayed semantic-syntactic impairments (and in some cases also phonological impairments), whereas 13 subjects had phonological impairments alone (mild to moderate in severity). When the subjects were reexamined in the first grade, 46% were found to be poor readers (i.e., performance ≥ 1 SD below the mean of a control group on tests of word identification and word attack). Consistent with previous findings, only a small percentage of the children with phonological disorders alone had reading problems (15%). Reading difficulties were much more prevalent among those who had displayed semantic-syntactic impairments in kindergarten (61%). Further analyses indicated that the type of semantic-syntactic deficit (i.e., receptive or expressive) did not appear to be related to reading outcome and that the severity of the language impairment showed only a low to moderate correlation with reading. The best predictor of reading outcome proved to be a measure of phonological awareness. Phonological awareness refers to children's explicit awareness of the speech sound structure of language. Catts et al. (1991) found that, among the speech-language–impaired children, the subjects who became good readers consistently performed better than the others on a kindergarten task involving the production of a word after deleting an initial syllable or phoneme.

Magnusson and Naucler (1990) have also reported phonological awareness to be a good predictor of academic success in LI children. They examined 37 LI and 37 matched control subjects 1 year before starting school, at the beginning of first grade, and at the end of first grade. Although, as a group, the LI children were found to be poorer readers at the end of first grade than the control subjects, some of the LI subjects actually were better readers than their matched control subjects. What these good readers had in common with other good students was high performance on tasks measuring the subject's awareness of the speech sounds in words.

Other investigators, examining a wider cross-section of children (as opposed to only LI children), have also found a strong relationship between phonological awareness and reading development/disorders (Bradley & Bryant, 1985; Stanovich, Cunningham, & Cramer, 1984; Treiman & Baron, 1981). This work is part of a larger body of research that indicates that certain deficits in the phonological domain are closely linked with reading disabilities (Catts, 1989a, 1989b; Stanovich, 1988). This research will be briefly reviewed below. For a more detailed discussion, see Catts (1989b) and Wagner and Torgesen (1987).

PHONOLOGICAL PROCESSING AND READING DISABILITIES

Numerous investigations conducted during the last 10 to 15 years have begun to converge and now demonstrate a relationship between what are termed phonological processing deficits and reading disorders. This research has focused on phonology or phonological processing from a somewhat different perspective than the one traditionally taken in speech-language pathology and related fields. The latter disciplines have generally examined phonology in terms of children's ability to produce accurately the sound segments of speech. As noted above, measurements of this ability have not generally been shown to be related to reading development. Recently, however, researchers have investigated other aspects of phonological processing in relationship to reading (Catts, 1989b; Liberman & Shankweiler, 1985; Wagner & Torgesen, 1987). This work has found a close link between reading disabilities and deficits in phonological awareness, problems in the retrieval of phonological information (i.e., word-finding problems), and deficits in the use of phonological codes in verbal memory.

Phonological awareness deficits

As noted above, many recent studies have reported a relationship between reading achievement and the awareness of the sound structure of spoken words. Poor readers, compared to good readers, have generally been shown to be less aware or sensitive to the speech sounds in words.

Poor readers, compared to good readers, have generally been shown to be less aware or sensitive to the speech sounds in words.

Reading group differences or correlations have been observed in tasks requiring children (1) to detect words that rhyme or begin/end with the same sounds (Bradley & Bryant, 1985), (2) to count the number of phonemes or syllables in words (Lundberg, 1982; Pratt & Brady, 1988), (3) to pronounce a word after deleting an initial or final segment (Fox & Routh, 1980; Kamhi & Catts, 1986; Lencher, Gerber, & Routh, 1990), and (4) to compare the length of spoken words (Katz, 1986; Pratt & Brady, 1988). The relationship between reading problems and poor phonological awareness can be explained, in part, on the basis of the poor readers' lack of experience in reading an alphabetic language (see Catts, 1989b). It is argued that learning to read an alphabetic language specifically highlights the phonemic structure of words. Thus individuals who are less skilled in using an alphabetic language would be expected to have less awareness of the individual phonemes in words.

Whereas reading may influence phonological awareness, phonological awareness also appears to affect reading. Research demonstrates that some aspects of speech sound awareness (e.g., awareness of rhyme or syllables) are acquired before formal reading instruction and that differences in this awareness influence reading development. For example, Share, Jorm, MacLean, and Mathews (1984), Stanovich et al. (1984), Lundberg, Olofssen, and Wall (1980), and Mann and Liberman (1984) have reported that measures of phonological awareness in kindergarten are strong predictors of reading ability in first grade. Bradley and Bryant (1985) and Maclean, Bryant, and Bradley (1987) have further observed that individual differences in

phonological awareness among children 3 to 5 years of age correlate significantly with their later reading ability. These studies, as well as those discussed above (Catts, 1991; Magnusson & Naucler, 1990), suggest that poor phonological awareness in the preschool and kindergarten years may be an early indicator of a reading disability.

Word retrieval problems

A related body of literature indicates that poor readers or children at risk for reading problems often have difficulties retrieving phonological information from memory (Wolf, 1984). Clinical observations have shown that these children frequently have word-finding difficulties and sometimes are described as dysnomic (e.g., Rudel, 1985). Naming problems in poor readers also have been documented in research. Wolf (1982), for example, has reported that poor readers have significant problems recalling the names of pictured objects on the Boston Naming Test. Because many of the objects that the poor readers failed to name were quite common and known to the subjects, Wolf (1982) concluded that these children's word-finding problems were due to difficulties in retrieving the sound codes or names of the objects from memory.

Poor readers also have been shown to perform less well than good readers on other tasks requiring name retrieval. For example, Denckla and Rudel (1976) reported that children with reading problems were slower than normal control subjects on rapid automatized naming (RAN) tasks. In these tasks, subjects are required to name five familiar symbols (involving letters, digits, colors, or objects) that are each randomly repeated 10 times on a 50-item stimulus card. More recently, Wolf and colleagues (Wolf, 1984, 1986; Wolf, Bally, & Morris, 1985) have extended the work of Denckla and Rudel (1976). In a longitudinal investigation, these researchers examined rapid naming ability (RAN and other similar tasks) and various aspects of reading ability in 115 children at the end of kindergarten, first grade, and second grade. Their results showed that rapid naming tasks given in kindergarten were good predictors of reading achievement in the primary grades. Children who performed poorly on these tasks in kindergarten were generally among the poorest readers at the end of second grade. Most recently, Catts (1991) and Felton and Brown (1989) also have found that rapid naming tasks administered in kindergarten are predictive of reading problems in at-risk populations.

Verbal memory deficits

Poor readers also have been shown to have problems in verbal short-term memory (Torgesen, 1985). Research indicates that poor readers perform less well than good readers in the short-term recall of digits, word strings, and sentences (Mann, Liberman, & Shankweiler, 1980; Shankweiler, Liberman, Mark, Fowler, & Fischer, 1972). In addition, measurements of verbal short-term memory in kindergarten have been found to be predictive of reading ability in first grade (Mann & Liberman, 1984). Whereas memory problems in poor readers may be explained in part on the basis of inefficient use of memory strategies, these problems also appear to be a direct result of phonological processing deficits (Torgesen, 1985). Specifically,

it is argued that poor readers have problems in using phonological codes to maintain verbal information in memory (Catts, 1989b; Wagner & Torgesen, 1987).

Another example of poor readers' problems in using phonological memory codes may be the difficulties that these children display in learning to pronounce new words in their oral vocabulary. Poor readers often misarticulate newly learned words, especially multisyllabic words (Miles, 1983). The production of these words often includes substitutions or transpositions of phonemes or the use of malapropisms. In a recent investigation, Kamhi, Catts, and Mauer (1990) found that poor readers took longer and made more errors than good readers in learning to pronounce the names (pseudowords) of four novel objects. On the basis of both production and recognition data, the authors concluded that the poor readers' speech production problems were due, at least in part, to difficulties in developing phonological representations in memory (also see Snowling, Goulandris, Bowlby, & Howell, 1985).

Poor readers' problems in producing multisyllabic words may, however, go beyond encoding deficits. Recently, Catts (1986, 1989c) found that poor readers also have problems in producing familiar but phonologically complex words and phrases (e.g., *animal, cinnamon,* and *sea shells*). It was concluded that the phonological processing deficits of poor readers extends to difficulties in programming sound sequences during the planning stages of speech production (also see Wolf, Michel, & Ovurt, 1990). Miles (1983) and Slingerland (1970) have observed similar deficits and have included stimulus items to assess these problems in their tests of reading/learning disabilities.

IMPLICATIONS FOR EARLY IDENTIFICATION

It should be clear from the above discussion that a reading disability is much more than a problem with recognizing and making sense of written language. It appears to be a more extensive disorder that is present well before children are confronted with formal reading instruction. In fact, in many cases, the disorder is better described as a developmental language disability that interferes with the acquisition of spoken and written language. Not only is this description more comprehensive, but it provides the necessary framework for early identification. According to this view, the disorder involves a developmental course of language problems that begins before school entry and reading failure.

Thus the presence of these language problems during the preschool years may serve as evidence for the early identification of reading disabilities. It is important to note, however, that in this conceptualization of the problem early language difficulties are not necessarily seen as being causally related to later reading difficulties. That is, naming deficits or syntactic problems, for example, may not directly cause difficulties in learning to read. Rather, it is proposed that preschool language problems and reading disabilities are each manifestations of a linguistic processing limitation(s) that underlies the disorder (Catts, 1989a; Kamhi & Catts, 1989).

Research reviewed in this article sug-gests that various oral language problems may precede and foretell reading disabilities. Numerous studies indicate that delays or deficits in the development of the semantic-syntactic aspects of language may be early indicators of a potential reading disability. Preschool children displaying these early language problems more often have reading difficulties upon entering school than normally developing children or children with articulation/phonological problems alone. The specific nature of these semantic-syntactic deficits and their relationship to reading problems, however, is still somewhat unclear. Thus far, research has failed to find a consistent relationship between the severity or type (receptive or expressive) of language impairment and reading outcome. In regard to severity, Scarborough (1991) has suggested that it is the presence of preschool language problems that is the crucial factor and that variability in reading outcome may be explained by other biological and/or environmental factors that influence reading achievement. Given the numerous variables that may have an impact on early reading acquisition, this conclusion seems reasonable. Nevertheless, firm conclusions in this regard should await further investigation. As studies specifically examine the relationship between type and severity of preschool language impairment and reading disabilities, and

Research reviewed in this article suggests that various oral language problems may precede and foretell reading disabilities.

as the relevant variables (e.g., age of the LI children, type of reading problems, and sensitivity of language measures) are better controlled, we will be able to draw more accurate conclusions for early identification purposes.

Beyond semantic-syntactic problems, research has shown a strong connection between reading disabilities and phonological processing deficits. As reviewed above, a large body of research indicates that children at risk for reading disabilities have limited explicit awareness of the sound segments in words. Poor readers or children at risk for reading problems also have been shown to have difficulties in word finding or problems in retrieving phonological information. Deficits in verbal short-term memory also have been associated with reading disabilities. Children at risk for reading disabilities often show difficulties in remembering directions or messages or have problems with learning new words, particularly multisyllabic words. Some also may have difficulties in producing complex phonological sequences. Research suggests that each of these various deficits may be an early sign of a potential reading disability and, therefore, should be included in programs or tasks designed for the early identification of reading disabilities.

FUTURE CONSIDERATIONS

Although recent research has significantly advanced our understanding of the language basis of reading disabilities, much more work in this area is necessary to improve early identification. For example, most investigations of the language basis

of reading disorders (especially those in the area of phonological processing) have limited their analyses (or the reporting of their data) to group comparisons or regression procedures. Whereas group differences and estimates of explained variance are important, they do not provide a complete enough picture for early identification purposes (Badian, 1988). These results do not necessarily tell us the likelihood that a poor performance on one measure (e.g., phonological awareness) will be associated with a similarly poor performance on another measure (e.g., reading). Data from Bradley and Bryant (1985) illustrate this point. They reported a significant moderate correlation between a preschool sound awareness task and first grade reading achievement. This finding suggests that children who performed poorly on the sound awareness task also performed poorly in reading and that subjects who performed well on the phonological awareness task scored well in reading. When extreme scores were observed, however, Bradley and Bryant (1985) found that their sound awareness measure was a better predictor for subjects who did well on this task than for those who did poorly (also see Mann, 1986). Although this result was based on a small sample and was only the case for preschool children and not kindergarten children, it illustrates the need for analyses that focus on the accuracy (e.g., hit or miss rate) or criterion discrimination of language measures in predicting reading achievement.

Also relevant to early identification is the question of the specificity of the language problems associated with reading disabilities. That is, it is important to know whether each of the various language deficits discussed above is directly related to reading development/disorders or whether some language problems are more central to reading than others. Some researchers have proposed that phonological processing deficits (Catts, 1989a; Jorm & Share, 1983; Liberman & Shankweiler, 1985) or even, more specifically, problems in phonological awareness (Pennington, 1989; Stanovich, 1988) are more closely related to reading difficulties than semantic-syntactic language problems. According to this view, semantic-syntactic deficits are correlated problems that often occur together with a reading disability but are not central to the disability. This proposal is based on clinical observations and limited research (Kamhi & Catts, 1986; Kamhi, Catts, Mauer, Apel, & Gentry, 1989), which suggest that many poor readers have no history of semantic-syntactic problems but do have difficulties in phonological processing/awareness. Most recently, this proposal has been challenged by Scarborough (1990), who, as reported earlier, found a strong relationship between early syntactic problems and later reading disabilities. Are these problems evidence for a more general language disability underlying reading disabilities, or do they suggest that the core deficit should be expanded to include some syntactic problems (perhaps subtle ones) but not others? Future research will need to address this issue.

The above discussion underscores the need for more research in general concerning the identification of reading disabilities. Although preschool language difficulties appear to be good predictors of later reading problems, research will also need to look beyond language factors. Language factors by no means explain all the variance in reading development or account for all cases of reading disabilities. Reading is a complex cognitive activity, and as such it is influenced by biological factors other than language ability (e.g., visual processing abilities) as well as numerous environmental factors (e.g., early literacy experience). These factors will need to be considered in combination with language variables to improve the early identification of reading disabilities.

---

*This article focuses primarily on the early identification of specific reading disabilities. For ease of reference, however, the term *reading disabilities* is used interchangeably with *specific reading disabilities*. The specificity of reading disabilities is currently a topic of much debate. Some researchers have argued that specific and nonspecific reading disabilities may be similar in their underlying causes (Siegel, 1989; Stanovich, 1988). Therefore, these disabilities may be identified on the basis of similar variables. Because of space limitations, a more extensive discussion of this issue is beyond the scope of the present article.

REFERENCES

Aaron, P. (1989). *Dyslexia and hyperlexia: Diagnosis and management of developmental reading disabilities.* Boston: Kluwer.

Aram, D., & Hall, N. (1989). Longitudinal follow-up of children with preschool communication disorders: Treatment implications. *School Psychology Review, 18,* 487–501.

Aram, D., & Nation, J. (1980). Preschool language disorders and subsequent language and academic difficulties. *Journal of Communication Disorders, 13,* 159–179.

Badian, N. (1988). Predicting dyslexia in a preschool population. In R. Masland & M. Masland (Eds.), *Preschool prediction of reading failure* (pp. 78–106). Parkton, MD: York.

Bishop, D., & Adams, C. (1990). A prospective study of the relationship between specific language impairment, phonological disorders and reading retardation. *Journal of Child Psychology and Psychiatry, 31,* 1027–1050.

Bishop, D., & Edmundson, A. (1987). Language impaired 4-year olds: Distinguishing transient from persistent impairment. *Journal of Speech and Hearing Disorders, 52,* 156–173.

Bradley, L., & Bryant, P. (1985). *Rhyme and reason in reading and spelling* (International Academy for Research in Learning Disabilities Monograph Series, No. 1). Ann Arbor, MI: University of Michigan Press.

Catts, H. (1986). Speech production/phonological deficits in reading disordered children. *Journal of Learning Disabilities, 19,* 504–508.

Catts, H. (1989a). Defining dyslexia as a developmental language disorder. *Annals of Dyslexia, 39,* 50–64.

Catts, H. (1989b). Phonological processing deficits and reading disabilities. In A. Kamhi and H. Catts (Eds.), *Reading disabilities: A developmental language perspective.* Austin, TX: Pro-ed.

Catts, H. (1989c). Speech production deficits in developmental dyslexia. *Journal of Speech and Hearing Disorders, 54,* 422–428.

Catts, H. (1991). Early identification of dyslexia: Evidence of a follow-up study of speech-language impaired children. *Annals of Dyslexia, 41.*

Chasty, H. (1985). What is dyslexia? A developmental language perspective. In M. Snowling (Ed.), *Children's written language difficulties: Assessment and management* (pp. 11–28). Windsor, England: NFER-Nelson.

Critchely, M. (1970). *The dyslexic child.* Springfield, IL: Thomas.

Denckla, M., & Rudel, R. (1976). Rapid automatized naming (RAN): Dyslexia differentiated from other learning disabilities. *Neuropsychologia, 14,* 471–479.

Doehring, D., Trites, R., Patel, P., & Fiederowicz, C. (1981). *Reading disabilities: The interaction of reading, language, and neuropsychological deficits.* New York: Academic Press.

Donahue, M. (1984). Learning disabled children's comprehension and production of syntactic devices for marking given versus new information. *Applied Psycholinguistics, 5,* 101–116.

Donahue, M. (1986). Linguistic and communicative development in learning disabled children. In S. Ceci (Ed.), *Handbook of cognitive, social, and neuro-psychological aspects of learning disabilities* (pp. 262–289). Hillsdale, NJ: Erlbaum.

Feagans, L., & Short, E. (1984). Developmental differences in the comprehension and production of narratives by reading disabled and normally achieving children. *Child Development, 55,* 1727–1736.

Felton, R., & Brown, I. (1989). Phonological processes as predictors of specific reading skills in children at risk for reading failures. *Reading and Writing: An Interdisciplinary Journal, 2,* 3–23.

Fletcher, J., Satz, P., & Scholes, R. (1981). Developmental changes in the linguistic performance correlates of reading achievement. *Brain and Language, 13,* 78–90.

Fox, B., & Routh, D. (1980). Phonemic analysis and severe reading disability. *Journal of Psycholinguistic Research, 9,* 115–119.

Hall, P., & Tomblin, J. (1978). A follow-up study of children with articulation and language disorders. *Journal of Speech and Hearing Disorders, 43,* 227–241.

Hessler, G. (1987). Educational issues surrounding severe discrepancy. *Learning Disabilities Research, 3,* 43–49.

Ingram, T., Mason, M., & Blackburn, I. (1970). A retrospective study of 82 children with reading disabilities. *Developmental Medical Child Neurology, 12,* 271–281.

Jansky, J., & De Hirsch, K. (1972). *Preventing reading failure—Prediction, diagnosis, intervention.* New York: Harper & Row.

Johnston, P., & Winograd, P. (1985). Passive failure in reading. *Journal of Reading Behavior, 17,* 279–301.

Jorm, A., & Share, D. (1983). Phonological recoding and reading acquisition. *Applied Psycholinguistics, 4,* 103–147.

Kamhi, A., & Catts, H. (1986). Toward an understanding of developmental language and reading disorders. *Journal of Speech and Hearing Disorders, 51,* 337–347.

Kamhi, A., & Catts, H. (1989). *Reading disabilities: A developmental language perspective.* Austin, TX: Pro-ed.

Kamhi, A., Catts, H., & Mauer, D. (1990). Explaining speech production errors in poor readers. *Journal of Learning Disabilities, 23,* 632–636.

Kamhi, A., Catts, H., Mauer, D., Apel, K., & Gentry, B. (1989). Phonological and spatial processing abilities in language- and reading-impaired children. *Journal of Speech and Hearing Disorders, 53,* 316–327.

Katz, R. (1986). Phonological deficiencies in children with reading disability: Evidence from an object-naming task. *Cognition, 22,* 225–257.

Lencher, O., Gerber, M., & Routh, D. (1990). Phonological awareness tasks as predictors of decoding ability: Beyond segmentation: *Journal of Learning Disabilities, 23,* 240–247.

Levi, G., Capozzi, F., Fabrizi, A., & Sechi, E. (1982). Language disorders and prognosis for reading disabilities in developmental age. *Perceptual and Motor Skills, 54,* 1119–1122.

Liberman, I., & Shankweiler, D. (1985). Phonology and the problems of learning to read and write. *Remedial and Special Education, 6,* 8–17.

Lundberg, I. (1982). Linguistic awareness as related to dyslexia. In Y. Zotterman (Ed.), *Dyslexia: Neuronal, Cognitive and Linguistic Aspects,* New York: Pergamon.

Lundberg, I., Olofssen, A., & Wall, S. (1980). Reading and spelling skills in the first school years, predicted from phonemic awareness skills in kindergarten. *Scandinavian Journal of Psychology, 21*, 59–173.

Maclean, M., Bryant, P., & Bradley, L. (1987). Rhymes, nursery rhymes, and reading in early childhood. *Merrill-Palmer Quarterly, 33*, 255–281.

Magnusson, E., & Naucler, K. (1990). Reading and spelling in language-disordered children—Linguistic and metalinguistic prerequisites: Report on a longitudinal study. *Clinical Linguistics and Phonetics, 4*, 49–61.

Mann, V. (1986). Why some children encounter reading problems: The contribution of difficulties with language processing and phonological sophistication to early reading disability. In J. Torgesen and B. Wong (Eds.), *Psychological and educational perspectives on learning disabilities* (pp. 133–161). New York: Academic Press.

Mann, V., & Liberman, I. (1984). Phonological awareness and verbal short-term memory. *Journal of Learning Disabilities, 17*, 592–599.

Mann V., Liberman, I., & Shankweiler, D. (1980). Children's memory for sentences and word strings in relation to reading ability. *Memory and Cognition, 8*, 329–335.

Masland, R., & Masland, M. (1988). *Preschool prevention of reading failure.* Parkton, MD: York.

Miles, T. (1983). *Dyslexia: The pattern of difficulties.* Springfield, IL: Thomas.

Miller, J., & Chapman, R. (1981). *Assessing language production in children.* Baltimore: University Park Press.

Pennington, B. (1989). Using genetics to understand dyslexia. *Annals of Dyslexia, 39*, 81–93.

Pratt, A., & Brady, S. (1988). The relationship of phonological awareness to reading disability in children and adults. *Journal of Educational Psychology, 80*, 319–323.

Roth, F., & Spekman, N. (1989a). Higher-order language processes and reading disabilities. In A. Kamhi and H. Catts (Eds.), *Reading disabilities: A developmental language perspective.* Austin, TX: Pro-Ed.

Roth, F., & Spekman, N. (1989b). The oral syntactic proficiency of learning disabled students: A spontaneous story sampling analysis. *Journal of Speech and Hearing Research, 32*, 67–77.

Rudel, R. (1985). The definition of dyslexia: Language and motor deficits. In F. Duffy and N. Geschwind (Eds.), *Dyslexia: A neuroscientific approach to clinical evaluation* (pp. 33–54). Boston: Little, Brown.

Scarborough, H. (1990). Very early language deficits in dyslexic children. *Child Development, 61*, 1728–1743.

Scarborough, H. (1991). Early syntactic development of dyslexic children. *Annals of Dyslexia, 41*.

Seidenberg, P., & Berstein, D. (1986). The comprehension of similes and metaphors by learning disabled and nonlearning disabled children. *Language, Speech, and Hearing Services in Schools, 17*, 219–229.

Shankweiler, D., Liberman, I., Mark, L., Fowler, C., & Fischer, F. (1972). The speech code and learning to read. *Journal of Experimental Psychology: Human Learning and Memory, 5*, 531–545.

Share, D., Jorm, A., MacLean, R., & Mathews, R. (1984). Sources of individual differences in reading acquisition. *Journal of Educational Psychology, 76*, 1309–1324.

Shriberg, L., & Kwiatkowski, J. (1988). A follow-up study of children with phonologic disorders of unknown origin. *Journal of Speech and Hearing Disorders, 53*, 144–156.

Short, E., & Ryan, E. (1984). Metacognitive differences between skilled and less skilled readers: Remediating deficits through story grammar and attribution training. *Journal of Educational Psychology, 76*, 225–235.

Siegel, L. (1989). IQ is irrelevant to the definition of learning disabilities. *Journal of Learning Disabilities, 22*, 469–478.

Silva, P., McGee, R., & Williams, S. (1987). A longitudinal study of children with developmental language delay at age three: Later intelligence, reading, and behavior problems. *Developmental Medicine and Child Neurology, 29*, 630–640.

Slingerland, B. (1970). *Slingerland screening tests for identifying children with specific language disability.* Cambridge, MA: Educators Publishing Service.

Snowling, M., Goulandris, N., Bowlby, M., & Howell, P. (1985). Segmentation and speech perception in relation to reading skill: A developmental analysis. *Journal of Experimental Child Psychology, 41*, 489–507.

Stanovich, K. (1986). Matthew effects in reading: Some consequences of individual differences in the acquisition of literacy. *Reading Research Quarterly, 20*, 360–406.

Stanovich, K. (1988). The right and the wrong places to look for the cognitive locus of reading disability. *Annals of Dyslexia, 38*, 154–180.

Stanovich, K. (1991). Discrepancy definitions of reading disability: Has intelligence led us astray? *Reading Research Quarterly, 26*, 7–29.

Stanovich, K., Cunningham, A., & Cramer, B. (1984). Assessing phonological awareness in kindergarten children: Issues of task comparability. *Journal of Experimental Child Psychology, 38*, 175–190.

Stark, R., Bernstein, L., Condino, R., Bender, M., Tallal, P., & Catts, H. (1984). Four-year follow-up study of language impaired children. *Annals of Dyslexia, 34*, 49–68.

Tallal, P., Curtiss, S., & Kaplan, R. (1989). *The San Diego longitudinal study: Evaluating the outcomes of preschool impairment in language development.* Final report, National Institute of Neurological and Communicative Disorders and Stroke.

Torgesen, J. (1985). Memory processes in reading disordered children. *Journal of Learning Disabilities, 18*, 350–357.

Treiman, R., & Baron, J. (1981). Segmental analysis ability: Development and relation to reading ability. In G. Mackinnon & T. Waller (Eds.), *Reading research: Advances in theory and practice*. New York: Academic Press.

Vellutino, F. (1979). *Dyslexia: Theory and research*. Cambridge, MA: MIT Press.

Vogel, S. (1974). Syntactic abilities in normal and dyslexic children. *Journal of Learning Disabilities, 7*, 103–109.

Wagner, R., & Torgesen, J. (1987). The nature of phonological processing and its causal role in the acquisition of reading skills. *Psychological Bulletin, 101*, 192–212.

Weiner, P. (1985). The value of follow-up studies. *Topics in Language Disorders, 5*(3), 78–92.

Wilson, B., & Risucci, D. (1988). The early identification of developmental language disorders and the prediction of the acquisition of reading skills. In R. Masland and M. Masland (Eds.), *Preschool prevention of reading failure*. Parkton, MD: York.

Wolf, M. (1982). The word-retrieval process and reading in children and aphasics. In K. Nelson (Ed.), *Children's language* (Vol. 3, pp. 437–493). New York: Gardner.

Wolf, M. (1984). Naming, reading, and the dyslexias: A longitudinal overview. *Annals of Dyslexia, 34*, 87–136.

Wolf, M. (1986). Rapid alternating stimulus naming in the developmental dyslexias. *Brain and Language, 27*, 360–379.

Wolf, M., Bally, H., & Morris, R. (1985). Automaticity, retrieval processes, and reading: A longitudinal study in average and impaired readers. *Child Development, 57*, 988–1000.

Wolf, M., & Obregon, M. (1989). *88 children in search of a name: A five year investigation of rate, word-retrieval, and vocabulary in reading development and dyslexia*. Paper presented at the meeting of the Society for Research in Child Development, Kansas City, MO.

Wolf, P., Michel, G., & Ovurt, M. (1990). The timing of syllable repetitions in developmental dyslexia. *Journal of Speech and Hearing Research, 33*, 281–289.

Planning an assessment of listening and reading comprehension

Joanne F. Carlisle, PhD
Learning Disabilities Program
Department of Communication Sciences
and Disorders
Northwestern University
Evanston, Illinois

COMPARISONS of discourse comprehension through listening and reading can help diagnosticians and teachers determine why students have difficulties in understanding their textbooks or why they perform poorly on standardized tests of reading comprehension. Not many standardized norm-referenced tests provide a way to compare listening and reading comprehension, and the ones that do generally contain short passages. Practitioners may learn more about discourse comprehension by using informal reading inventories or by developing an informal or a curriculum-based measure of discourse comprehension.

This article discusses issues of concern to those who wish to assess comprehension of extended discourse. Toward this end, the first section discusses what can be learned about comprehension problems by assessment of discourse through listening and reading. The second section reviews developmental aspects of the relationship between listening and reading

Top Lang Disord, 1991,12(1),17–31
© 1991 Aspen Publishers, Inc.

comprehension skills. The third section discusses problems associated with selecting text passages and methods of testing comprehension. The final section describes the development of a set of passages and an accompanying sentence-verification test, illustrating how two students with different types of reading comprehension problems performed on the tests.

COMPARISONS OF LISTENING AND READING COMPREHENSION

The most common view of reading comprehension is the unitary view, which holds that the same comprehension processing takes place in reading and listening (see Danks, 1980; Sticht, 1979). According to this perspective, reading and listening differ in the modality of presentation (an auditory or a visual signal). Once encoding has taken place, however, the cognitive components of comprehension processing are essentially the same (Danks & End, 1987; Sinatra, 1990). The nature of, or problems related to, the encoding may have a considerable impact on comprehension processing in listening or reading. For example, a student who has difficulties with efficient auditory processing may not perform well on a listening comprehension test because he or she is unable to keep abreast of the speaker's rate of delivery. Unlike the text in reading, oral discourse is transitory and must be processed as it is presented. As a result, this same student may perform better on a reading comprehension test because he or she can read at his or her own pace. Conversely, a student who has word recognition problems may not be able to understand passages through reading as well as he or she can through listening. In reading, encoding linguistic information entails word recognition skills that are accurate and rapid enough that the processing of words and sentences is not impeded (Perfetti & Roth, 1981).

Among individuals with seemingly good comprehension capabilities, some may be better at listening than at reading and others may be better at reading than at listening. For example, Daneman and Carpenter (1980) have found some college students with better working memories for orally presented words and some with better working memories for visually presented words; these students usually had corresponding strengths in either listening to or reading text passages. Somewhat similarly, Carlisle and Felbinger (in press) have found that some of the fourth, fifth, and eighth graders in the regular classes that they tested were significantly weaker than their peers in listening than in reading, whereas others were significantly weaker in reading than in listening.

Among the students who do poorly on tests of reading comprehension relative to their peers, two kinds of comprehension difficulties are commonly found. One is a specific reading disability. This is suggested when listening is age appropriate and when reading comprehension performance is significantly weaker than listening. Follow-up testing usually indicates that such students have slow or inaccurate word recognition skills. The attention and time it takes for them to identify words make it difficult for them to use their otherwise adequate language comprehension processes effectively. Thus, although such students' scores on reading comprehension measures make them look as though they have comprehension problems, they actually have word recognition problems that impede their ability to understand written texts.

The second type of comprehension difficulty is a general comprehension problem, which is suggested by performances in both reading and listening comprehension that are significantly below grade-level expectations. Problems in linguistic or cognitive development might be suspected, and further testing in these areas is indicated. On a test of listening and reading comprehension, therefore, the main difference between the student with a specific reading disability and the student with a general language disability is usually the proficiency of his or her listening comprehension.

Students with these two types of problems may have similarly poor levels of performance on reading comprehension tests, so that their problems are not distinguished unless further testing is carried out. Both appear in unsorted groups of reading-disabled students in research studies as well as in classrooms (Rispens, 1990).

It seems clear that the two types of reading comprehension problems could be distinguished if a combination of listening comprehension, reading comprehension, and word recognition tests was used (Carlisle, 1989; Sticht & James, 1984). This method of identification has been explored by Aaron, Kuchta, and Grapenthin (1988). They gave a group of 38 reading-disabled children in grades 4 through 8 a listening comprehension test. Some of these students had normal listening performances. Further testing showed that these stu-

dents lacked knowledge of letter-sound correspondences but that they did not do poorly on various comprehension activities. Thus their problem with reading comprehension seemed to be attributable to insufficient skill in word recognition, which in turn held back their processing of the ideas. Another group of the students had poor listening performances. Unlike the specifically poor readers, these students had trouble with various comprehension activities. Thus they were experiencing difficulties with language comprehension that affected their performances in both modalities.

The results of this study illustrate that assessing reading comprehension, listening comprehension, and word recognition might be a viable way to begin to sort out significantly different types of reading problems. Correct identification is important because of the implications for designing appropriate instruction. For example, for the specifically disabled student, a primary focus in remediation is generally word recognition skills. For students with general language comprehension problems, however, a program of instruction in language comprehension would probably be indicated, pending the results of a full diagnostic assessment of language and cognitive capabilities.

Practitioners interested in determining

Practitioners interested in determining the nature of their students' comprehension problems must face the problem of how to carry out an appropriate assessment.

the nature of their students' comprehension problems must face the problem of how to carry out an appropriate assessment. Only a few standardized tests of reading and reading-related activities with current norms provide subtests of both listening and reading comprehension. Of the four tests most commonly used to assess reading for children who might qualify for Chapter 1 or special education services, according to a recent survey ("Survey reveals," 1991) only one—the Woodock-Johnson Psychoeducational Battery (WJPB)—contains subtests of both reading and listening comprehension. The WJPB subtests are made up of short passages and therefore do not require much in the way of text-processing strategies. Furthermore, the method of assessing comprehension (modified cloze procedure) places somewhat different demands on the student in listening than in reading (as will be discussed more fully later). Thus the subtests of the WJPB may not be a satisfactory means of carrying out direct comparison of listening and reading comprehension capabilities. Another survey of the diagnostic practices of reading and learning disabilities specialists suggests that tests of listening comprehension may not be used as a regular component in the diagnosis of reading disabilities (German, Johnson, & Schneider, 1985). Instead, the tests used by these specialists focus solely on components of reading (e.g., reading vocabulary, word attack skills, and oral reading).

What is needed is a method of assessing comprehension that provides a direct comparison of listening and reading comprehension and text passages that resemble fairly normal reading experiences. To meet these needs, tests other than norm-referenced standardized measures might be more helpful to gather information about students' discourse comprehension capabilities. One approach is to use one of the many published informal reading inventories (IRIs), which generally include a set of passages for assessing listening comprehension (see Jongsma & Jongsma, 1981). A second approach is to develop a curriculum-based measure of listening and reading comprehension (see Salvia & Hughes, 1990).

Curriculum-based assessment of listening and reading comprehension can be based on passages selected from the students' textbooks. Thus one advantage is that students are tested on the kinds of materials that they are expected to understand in their content-area courses. Such tests can also provide comparisons of normal and reading-disabled students in the same curriculum, and they can be used for pre- and post-testing. Thus the impact of different kinds of instruction or intervention can be assessed. In some situations, however, diagnosticians need to assess students who are not using the same textbooks or studying in the same classrooms. In such cases, an informal test may be devised by writing passages that are then tested to determine the level of readability (see Chall, 1984). Teachers may also be asked to rate the passages for their appropriateness for a given grade level.

Through one of these three systems—IRIs, curriculum-based measures, or informal tests of listening and reading comprehension—diagnosticians may get a better idea of their students' understanding of extended discourse than they would get through using most current standardized tests.

DEVELOPMENTAL CHANGES IN DISCOURSE COMPREHENSION

Interpretations of students' performances on tests of listening and reading comprehension must be carried out with an understanding of developmental changes in the relationship of listening and reading over the school years. Children are first exposed to a number of different kinds of discourse through listening. As they learn to read, they use these same capabilities to understand written texts. In their first years of school, students are usually better at understanding discourse through listening than through reading because their word-recognition skills are not proficient enough to allow them to read for themselves texts that they can understand through listening (Sticht & James, 1984). Thus first graders might read Dr. Seuss's *Hop on Pop* for themselves but can understand *Horton Hatches the Egg* only if it is read aloud to them. By about the fifth grade, most children have developed the facility in word recognition needed to read and understand texts comparable in difficulty to the ones that they understand through listening (Sticht & James, 1984).

Accuracy of word recognition is not sufficient. Children must be able to recognize the words in their texts fast enough that lexical access and other aspects of linguistic processing (assigning semantic and syntactic roles, for instance) can take

place in a timely manner. The integration of ideas within and across sentences is dependent on complete and efficient processing at basic linguistic levels. Slow processing may mean that undue attention needs to be devoted to lower-level processes, so that maintaining and integrating the ideas in working memory is impeded (Perfetti & Roth, 1981).

Other differences between listening and reading may cause some young students to have more trouble with reading than with listening comprehension. To some extent, the language structures used in written discourse differ from those used in oral discourse. Gradually, however, young students adjust to the language of written texts (Leu, 1982). In addition, some young readers have difficulty making up for the absence of prosodic cues in written texts. This, too, may make reading comprehension initially more difficult than listening comprehension (Mann, Cowin, & Schoenheimer, 1989; Schreiber & Read, 1980).

Students who experience severe and prolonged difficulties in learning to read may develop additional problems over time. Students with poor word-recognition skills either may not read much or may not read books as challenging as those their peers read. As a result, they may have less of an opportunity to develop their word and world knowledge to the same extent as their peers (Stanovich, 1986). They have increasing difficulty in understanding the types of texts they encounter in their courses because of gaps in their vocabulary and background knowledge. Such gaps also affect comprehension through listening. Thus, over time, such students may have increasingly poor performances on tests of both listening and reading comprehension relative to their peers. They then appear to have generally depressed comprehension capabilities instead of specific reading disabilities.

The changing relationship between listening and reading skills suggests two particular problems in assessing elementary school students. One problem stems from the fact that listening performance is usually better than reading performance. Sticht (1979) has proposed that a student's listening performance be used as an estimate of reading potential, that is, the level of comprehension that the student might be able to achieve were his or her word recognition skills more highly developed. Even in the elementary years, however, some students perform better on reading than on listening measures (Fletcher & Pumfrey, 1988). For this reason, it may be better to regard listening as a performance measure, not an index of potential for achievement in reading.

A second problem involves the assessment of silent reading in young students. For some, silent reading is not a familiar or effective means of carrying out a reading task. Oral reading could possibly be used in place of, or in addition to, silent reading. For example, Hinchley and Levy (1988) compared third and sixth graders' comprehension of passages after oral reading, silent reading, and listening. They found that at both grade levels silent reading and listening performances did not differ significantly but that comprehension after oral reading surpassed both. Oral reading may ensure closer attention to the text and for this reason may facilitate superior comprehension and recall.

DESIGNING A TEST TO COMPARE LISTENING AND READING

The usefulness of comparisons of listening and reading performances depends on the extent to which the passages used for reading and listening are appropriate and comparable in structure and level of difficulty. Assessing students with a type of discourse with which they have had little experience might result in misrepresentation of their comprehension capabilities. One study has shown mismatches in passages in basal readers and standardized tests, a situation that may affect students' test performances (Flood, Lapp, & Flood, 1984). In designing or choosing a means of assessing discourse comprehension, then, it is helpful to understand what constitutes appropriate choices of genre and text structure for children at different educational levels.

It is also important to think carefully about the task used to assess comprehension and recall. What students understand and remember from passages may be affected by what they are asked to do after reading or listening to passages. There are many ways to test comprehension and recall, but some are more appropriate for different purposes and different types of students than others.

Genre and text structure

When children start school, their experiences with different kinds of extended discourse are fairly limited. They are most familiar with anecdotes, explanations of events or simple phenomena, the running commentaries of their playmates, and narratives encountered in story-reading shared with adults. Preschool experiences with story reading, in particular, have been found to be strongly related to children's success in reading in their first few years in school (Wells, 1985). Once in school, they gradually become accustomed to different genres and functions of tests, including those encountered in the study of literature (poetry, biography, and drama) and the types of exposition used in science and social studies.

Even though students are gradually exposed to different kinds of expository texts, their comprehension of informational passages still lags behind their comprehension of narratives in the third grade (Rasool & Royer, 1986). This lag may reflect not only the relative amount of experience that they have had with the two kinds of discourse but also aspects of their cognitive development.

With all genres, most students gradually develop an awareness of structural relations and a capacity to use basic structures to understand and remember texts. In their understanding of stories, young children focus on actions and simple patterns of events. As they grow older, they see narratives in terms of underlying themes and purposes (Applebee, 1978; Stein & Glenn, 1979). In the same way that children gradually come to understand the common elements of narratives, they also gradually learn about the conventions of structure and expression associated with different types of expository texts. Researchers believe that awareness of text structures may be what facilitates their use as a means for understanding and remembering texts (Richgels, McGee, Lomax, & Sheard, 1987; Taylor & Samuels, 1983).

Some expository text structures are easier for students to understand than others because the logical relations among ideas vary in complexity (Horowitz, 1987; Meyer, 1984). In the list of text structures in Table 1, for example, enumeration generally entails coordination of information used to support the main idea, a simple listing of details or ideas of equal rank, whereas cause–effect entails understanding of antecedents and consequences. Thus in a passage listing kinds of snakes, the structure (enumeration) might help a young student remember the passage; in contrast, in a passage that explains why some kinds of snakes go for long periods of time without needing food, the structure (cause) might be too complex to aid comprehension and recall.

Table 1. Common text structures of expository passages

Type	Description
Enumeration	Series of facts or details related to a topic
Sequence	Series of events related in temporal order
Description	Specific attributes or characteristics of a topic
Comparison	Comparison/contrast of two or more topics or several aspects of one topic
Cause–effect	Antecedents and consequences; how one thing makes another happen
Problem–solution	Introduces remark and reply, question and answer, problem and solution formats

Younger students have been shown to perform less well on the more complex text structures than older students. For instance, Hinchley and Levy (1988) identified a group of third- and sixth-grade students who were insensitive to the structure of stories. Englert and Hiebert (1984) found that third graders were more likely to grasp sequences than descriptions. Older children (fifth and sixth grade) more consistently understand and use enumerative, sequence, and description structures; they may have some difficulty with comparisons and considerable difficulty with cause as a text structure (Richgels et al., 1987; Zinar, 1991).

Poor readers may have particular problems with comprehension of text structures. Englert and Thomas (1987) assessed learning-disabled students (all with significant reading problems), a group of reading age matched peers, and a group of same age peers (spanning grades 3 through 8) on their understanding and use of text structures. The learning-disabled students performed better on sequences of events than on comparisons, as we might expect. They were generally less sensitive to the different forms of expository structures than their reading age matched peers, however. Thus, although children gradually become wiser about the methods at their disposal for structuring, integrating, and effectively remembering ideas as they listen or read, students with serious reading disabilities may show less awareness of text structures than their peers.

The sequence of mastery of genre and text structure reviewed above presents some guidelines for developing or choosing a test of comprehension. First, at least up to the third grade, narrative passages might be the appropriate choice. Between about fourth grade and junior high school, the use of expository passages can help us judge whether the children are going to have trouble with their content area textbooks (e.g., history or science). It may be best to use relatively simple text structures, however (e.g., enumeration, sequence, or description). The more complex forms of discourse (e.g., comparison or cause) are most appropriate for able students at a junior high level or beyond.

Choosing an appropriate task

Because it is a receptive language process, comprehension is hard to assess. We must try to figure out what a child has understood in the least intrusive way possible. When we present children with a task through which we hope they will demonstrate their understanding of a text, we may unknowingly overburden their expressive language capabilities and end up believing they understood little. Alternatively, we may unknowingly provide guiding information about the meaning of the text (as, for example, in asking questions) and end up thinking they understood more than they did. In fact, different types of tasks may affect the way the student constructs meaning from the text.

Most standardized reading tests use multiple-choice questions. Children with good test-taking strategies benefit by the opportunity to eliminate some options and

Because it is a receptive language process, comprehension is hard to assess.

improve their chances of selecting correct answers. Learning-disabled children appear to lack the kinds of metacognitive skills that many of their nondisabled peers have (Davey, 1987). The use of open-ended questions, common on published IRIs, may be preferable. In some cases, these help us understand whether children have picked up particular pieces of information or even main ideas. Nonetheless, whether multiple-choice or open-ended questions are used, diagnosticians should be aware that the questions themselves may cause a child to reorganize his or her initial understanding of a text (Johnston, 1983). Thus the question "Why did Johnny hide the bat?" indicates that Johnny hid the bat, an event the child may not have understood until the question was asked.

Because of dissatisfaction with questions as a means of testing comprehension, other tasks have become popular in recent years. Free recall has regained popularity. Its validity has recently been investigated both as an oral and a written task (Fuchs, Fuchs, & Maxwell, 1988). This method may provide insight into the student's grasp of text structure, sequence of events, and so on. On the other hand, some students cannot demonstrate their full understanding or memory of discourse through free recall. Young students tend to give either short or rather scattered recalls. In fact, they can often provide details in answer to specific questions that they did not provide in retelling a story. Students with expressive language difficulties are put at a great disadvantage when asked to retell a story, as are students with attention deficits.

Cloze procedure is a third method commonly used to test comprehension. This method involves removing words at regular intervals from a text and evaluating the student's ability to provide an appropriate word for each omission. It is likely that cloze procedure best evaluates the ability to make sensible semantic and syntactic judgments (Kibby, 1981). Comprehension on the sentence level is assessed, whereas important aspects of discourse comprehension, such as the students' ability to grasp the text structure and to come to a sense of the overall meaning of the passage, may not be assessed (Kintsch & Yarbrough, 1982). An additional problem is that cloze procedure does not permit a direct comparison of comprehension processes through listening and reading. When cloze procedure is used with reading passages, the students can study the passage (including rereading parts or reading ahead in the passage) to decide on their answers. When cloze procedure is used with listening, the students cannot study the passage in the same way. They must have decided on an appropriate answer as they listen or else depend entirely on memory of the text to formulate an answer.

One other method for assessing comprehension is sentence verification. This method involves presenting the student with a passage to read or listen to. Without recourse to the passage, the student then indicates whether the idea in each test sentence was or was not in the original passage. Different kinds of test sentences can be devised to tap different types of language comprehension problems. A passage followed by four test sentences is given in the appendix. The types of test sentences used here were developed by Royer and colleagues (Royer, 1986). They include originals (sentences taken directly from the passage), paraphrases (sentences with the same meaning but shifts in word choice and word order), meaning changes (sentences that are like originals except for the substitution of one word), and distractors (sentences with information about the topic not mentioned in the passage). The student who has grasped the intended meaning of the author will respond "yes" to originals and paraphrases and "no" to meaning changes and distractors.

This method has the advantage of not requiring expressive language for a response. In addition, it offers a comparable means of assessing listening and reading. Research results have suggested that sentence verification is a valid measure of language comprehension and is sensitive to students' ability to formulate a mental representation of the meaning of a text passage, not just comprehension of individual sentences (Royer, 1986). Royer, Greene, and Sinatra (1987) have published guidelines for constructing sentence verification tests.

Other methods are available and might be selected for particular reasons. For instance, picture identification after reading or listening may also avoid expressive language difficulties. Nevertheless, some students have difficulty with picture interpretation or other aspects of nonverbal abilities. In addition, this method lends itself best to short passages and "picturable" events. It is not a particularly good means of assessing discourse comprehension overall.

Practitioners are advised to keep in mind the advantages and disadvantages of the different methods of assessing comprehension. The method that is selected should suit the students and the circumstances under which they are being tested. A 7-year-old child with no known problems of language development might respond well if asked to retell a story, whereas a teenager with word retrieval difficulties would not. It may be helpful to keep in mind that no two students come away from an experience of discourse comprehension with exactly the same understanding. Individual strengths and weaknesses in linguistic knowledge, background knowledge, and strategies play a role in the construction of meaning (Wilson & Anderson, 1986). In addition, children may have had different educational backgrounds, including differences in the extensiveness of their experience learning by listening or by reading. For this reason, interviews, observations, and discussions of texts may richly supplement the more typical types of comprehension assessment. Valencia and Pearson (1988) offer general guidelines for assessment of comprehension in classroom contexts.

AN INFORMAL TEST AND TWO CASE STUDIES

One way to argue for the value of assessing both listening and reading of comprehension is to illustrate what might be learned from such an assessment. For this purpose, the development of an informal test of listening and reading comprehension is described. Then the assessment profiles of two students are presented. The project used for this illustration involved the comparison of an eighth-grade reading-disabled group with a reading age matched sixth-grade class. The two groups had been given a standardized reading test, the Gates-MacGinitie Reading Test (MacGinitie, 1978), earlier in the school year. The reading specialist had also administered the Gray Oral Reading Test (Gray, 1967) and the Wide Range Achievement Test (WRAT), Reading Subtest (Jastak & Wilkinson, 1984) to the eighth graders as part of the process of determining appropriate forms of remediation for their reading problems.

A test of reading and listening comprehension was developed for use in this project. The following questions were useful in developing the test:

1. What is the purpose of the test?
2. Therefore, what reading behaviors are to be measured?
3. What kinds of passages are appropriate, given the purpose of the test and the students for whom it is intended?
4. What type of task will best suit the purpose of the evaluation and the students for whom it is intended?

For this project, the purpose was to compare students with similar levels of reading comprehension to determine whether they did or did not differ in listening comprehension. It was also hoped that information gathered by the researchers might be useful in suggesting the nature of the students' reading disabilities, so that decisions about further diagnostic assessment could be made. Because the purpose was to compare levels of performance in reading and listening comprehension, the behaviors of interest were students' comprehension and recall of information after reading or listening to passages of equivalent levels of difficulty. The students who were going to take the reading and listening test were at different grade levels and in different classrooms. At

the eighth-grade level, the students were not all taking the same courses or using the same textbooks. Because a curriculum-based test would not have been an appropriate measure in this case, an informal test was developed.

The passages were written with information from encyclopedias in the school library. Because the students were in the sixth and eighth grades, it was appropriate to use a test consisting of expository passages. The passages were on such generally familiar topics as animals (e.g., the octopus) or natural phenomena (e.g., tornadoes). The passage entitled "Crows" in the appendix was one of the passages developed for this project. The students read and listened to six passages, each one about 200 words in length. The passages ranged from third-grade to an eighth-grade readability level, as was deemed appropriate for students with a sixth-grade reading level.

The listening and reading passages were followed by sentence verification tests, based on the technique devised by Royer and colleagues (Royer, 1986; Royer et al., 1987). This task was chosen because it purports to assess language comprehension of extended discourse and because demands placed on the student are comparable for listening and reading.

The sixth graders' performances on the Gates-MacGinitie Reading Test and the experimental listening and reading subtests are given in Table 2 to provide a basis for evaluating two eighth graders' performances. At the start of the project, the teacher of these eighth-grade boys, Charlie and Mike, considered that they needed similar kinds of instruction, given their performances on the standardized tests.

Table 2. Comparison of two eighth-grade boys in a remedial reading class

Tests	Scores		
	Charlie	Mike	Sixth graders (n = 10)
Gates-MacGinitie Reading, Level E, Form 1			Level D, form I
Vocabulary	6.3	6.7	6.4
Comprehension	5.6	6.7	7.2
Gray Oral Reading Form A	7.8	6.9	
WRAT Reading	Beginning, grade 5	End, grade 4	
Experimental test of listening and reading comprehension			
Listening passages	97% correct	72% correct	88% correct
Reading passages	76% correct	66% correct	86% correct

Mike was slightly weaker than Charlie on word recognition (see the WRAT reading scores) and oral reading (see the Gray oral reading scores), but the boys were both working on word recognition skills as well as reading comprehension skills.

The boys' performances on the informal test of listening and reading suggest that there may be different reasons for their reading comprehension problems. On the reading passages their performances were quite similar, but on the listening passages they were distinctly different. Charlie did well on the listening passages. Thus it seemed likely that his comprehension problem was specific to reading and might be attributable to slow and/or inaccurate word recognition processes. In contrast, Mike did relatively poorly on both listening and reading passages. Mike appeared to have a more generalized language comprehension problem. Further information about their listening/reading behaviors came from an informal teacher evaluation form (rating scale of study habits and attitudes) completed for this project. Mike was characterized as having trouble following oral

directions and attending to tasks in class. Charlie was characterized as a slow worker who had trouble getting tests and homework papers done on time.

Although these boys' performances on the listening and reading test indicated different types of comprehension problems, further testing was needed. For Charlie, the most important component was a complete evaluation of his word recognition problems. Was he inaccurate or slow at reading words? Did he have particular difficulties with nonsense words or nonphonetic "sight" words? For Mike, further testing was needed to determine the nature and extent of his oral language comprehension difficulties—for example, tests of receptive vocabulary and sentence comprehension. Eventually, the boys' programs of remediation were revised to reflect their particular needs.

• • •

Not all students do poorly on tests of reading comprehension for the same reason. In some cases the primary difficulty is inefficient or inaccurate word recognition processes, and in others it is a more general language comprehension problem. Comparisons of comprehension of extended discourse after listening and reading can help determine the nature of reading comprehension problems. Therefore, thoughtful consideration needs to be given to the selection or development of test instruments. This includes determination of appropriate kinds of discourse and text structures, passage content, and task. Such careful planning is needed to ensure that students' performances will reveal the dimensions of their difficulties understanding extended discourse.

REFERENCES

Aaron, P.G., Kuchta, S., & Grapenthin, C.T. (1988). Is there a thing called dyslexia? *Annals of Dyslexia, 38,* 33–49.

Applebee, A.N. (1978). *The child's concept of story.* Chicago: University of Chicago Press.

Carlisle, J.F. (1989). Diagnosing comprehension deficits through listening and reading. *Annals of Dyslexia, 39,* 159–176.

Carlisle, J.F., & Felbinger, L. (in press). Profiles in listening and reading comprehension. *Journal of Educational Psychology.*

Chall, J.S. (1984). Readability and prose comprehension: Continuities and discontinuities. In J. Flood (Ed.), *Understanding reading comprehension* (pp. 233–246). Newark, DE: International Reading Association.

Daneman, M., & Carpenter, P.A. (1980). Individual differences in working memory and reading. *Journal of Verbal Learning and Verbal Behavior, 19,* 450–466.

Danks, J. (1980). Comprehension in listening and reading. Same or different? In J. Danks & K. Pezdek (Eds.), *Reading and understanding.* Newark, DE: International Reading Association.

Danks, J.H., & End, L.J. (1987). Processing strategies for listening and reading. In R. Horowitz & S.J. Samuels (Eds.), *Comprehending oral and written language.* New York: Academic Press.

Davey, B. (1987). Postpassage questions: Task and reader effects on comprehension and metacomprehension processes. *Journal of Reading Behavior, 19,* 261–283.

Englert, C.S., Hiebert, E. (1984). Children's developing awareness of text structures in expository materials. *Journal of Educational Psychology, 76,* 65–74.

Englert, C.S., & Thomas, C.C. (1987). Sensitivity to text structure in reading and writing: A comparison between learning disabled and nonlearning disabled students. *Learning Disability Quarterly, 10,* 106–111.

Fletcher, J., & Pumfrey, P.D. (1988). Differences in text comprehension amongst 7–8-year-old children. *School Psychology International, 9,* 133–145.

Flood, J., Lapp, D., & Flood, S. (1984). Types of writing found in early levels of basal reading programs: Preprimers through second grade readers. *Annals of Dyslexia, 34,* 241–256.

Fuchs, L.S., Fuchs, D., & Maxwell, L. (1988). The validity of informal reading comprehension measures. *Remedial and Special Education, 9,* 20–28.

German, D., Johnson, B., & Schneider, M. (1985). Learning disability versus reading disability: Survey of practitioners, diagnostic populations and test instruments. *Learning Disability Quarterly, 8,* 141–155.

Gray, W.S. (1967). *Gray oral reading tests.* New York: Bobbs-Merrill.

Hinchley, J., & Levy, B.A. (1988). Developmental and individual differences in reading comprehension. *Cognition and Instruction, 5,* 3–47.

Horowitz, R. (1987). Rhetorical structure in discourse processing. In R. Horowitz & S.J. Samuels (Eds.), *Comprehending oral and written language* (pp. 117–160). New York, NY: Academic Press.

Jastak, S., & Wilkinson, G.S. (1984). *The Wide Range Achievement Test—Revised.* Wilmington, DE: Jastak Associates.

Johnston, P.H. (1983). *Reading comprehension assessment: A cognitive basis.* Newark, DE: International Reading Association.

Jongsma, K., & Jongsma, E. (1981). Test review: Commercial informal reading inventories. *Reading Teacher, 34,* 697–705.

Kibby, M.W. (1981). Test review: The degrees of reading power. *Journal of Reading, 24,* 416–427.

Kintsch, W., & Yarbrough, J.C. (1982). Role of rhetorical structure in text comprehension. *Journal of Educational Psychology, 74,* 828–834.

Leu, D.J. (1982). Differences between oral and written discourse and the acquisition of reading proficiency. *Journal of Reading Behavior, 14,* 111–125.

MacGinitie, W.H. (1978). *Gates-MacGinitie reading tests* (2nd ed). Chicago: Riverside.

Mann, V.A., Cowin, E., & Schoenheimer, J. (1989). Phonological processing, language comprehension, and reading ability. *Journal of Learning Disabilities, 22*, 76–89.

Meyer, B.J.F. (1984). Organizational aspects of text: Effects on reading comprehension and applications for the classroom. In J. Flood (Ed.), *Promoting reading comprehension.* Newark, DE: International Reading Association.

Perfetti, C.A., & Roth, S.F. (1981). Some of the interactive processes in reading and their role in reading skill. In A.M. Lesgold & C.A. Perfetti (Eds.), *Interactive processes in reading* (pp. 269–297). Hillsdale, NJ: Lawrence Erlbaum.

Rasool, J.M., & Royer, J.M. (1986). Assessment of reading comprehension using the sentence verification technique: Evidence from narrative and descriptive texts. *Journal of Educational Research, 79*, 180–184.

Richgels, D.J., McGee, L.M., Lomax, R.G., & Sheard, C. (1987). Awareness of four text structures: Effects on recall of expository texts. *Reading Research Quarterly, 22*, 177–196.

Rispens, J. (1990). Comprehension problems in dyslexia. In D.A. Balota, G.B. Flores d'Arcais, & K. Rayner (Eds.), *Comprehension processes in reading* (pp. 603–620). Hillsdale, NJ: Lawrence Erlbaum.

Royer, J.M. (1986). *The sentence verification technique as a measure of comprehension: Validity, reliability, and practicality.* Unpublished manuscript, University of Massachusetts.

Royer, J.M., Greene, B.A., & Sinatra, G.M. (1987). The sentence verification technique: A practical procedure for testing comprehension. *Journal of Reading, 30*, 414–422.

Salvia, J., & Hughes, C. (1990). *Curriculum-based assessment: Testing what is taught.* New York: Macmillan.

Schreiber, P., & Read, C. (1980). Children's use of phonetic cues in spelling, parsing, and—maybe—reading. *Bulletin of the Orton Society, 30*, 209–224.

Sinatra, G.M. (1990). Convergence of listening and reading processing. *Reading Research Quarterly, 15*, 115–130.

Stanovich, K.E. (1986). Matthew effects in reading: Some consequences of individual differences in the acquisition of literacy. *Reading Research Quarterly, 21*, 360–407.

Stein, N., & Glenn, G. (1979). An analysis of story comprehension in elementary school children. In R. Freedle (Ed.), *New directions in discourse processing* (Vol. 2, pp. 32–120). Norwood, NJ: Ablex.

Sticht, T. (1979). Applications of the Audread model to reading evaluation and instruction. In L.B. Resnick & P.A. Weaver (Eds.), *Theory and practice of early reading* (Vol. 1, pp. 209–226). Hillsdale, NJ: Lawrence Erlbaum.

Sticht, T.G., & James, H.J. (1984). Listening and reading. In P.D. Pearson (Ed.), *Handbook of reading research* (pp. 293–317). New York: Longman.

Survey reveals problems with diagnostic assessment. (1991, February). *Reading Today, 8*, 7.

Taylor, B., & Samuels, S.J. (1983). Children's use of text structures in the recall of expository material. *American Educational Research Journal, 20*, 517–528.

Valencia, S.W., & Pearson, P.D. (1988). Principles of classroom comprehension assessment. *Remedial and Special Education, 9*, 26–35.

Wells, G. (1985). Preschool literacy-related activities and success in school. In D.R. Olson, N. Torrance, & A. Hildyard (Eds.), *Literary, language, and learning: The nature and consequences of reading and writing* (pp. 229–255). Cambridge, MA: Cambridge University Press.

Wilson, P.T., & Anderson, R.C. (1986). What they don't know will hurt them: The role of prior knowledge in comprehension. In J. Orsanu (Ed.), *Reading comprehension: From research to practice* (pp. 31–48). Hillsdale, NJ: Lawrence Erlbaum.

Zinar, S. (1991). Fifth-graders' recall of prepositional content and causal relationships from expository prose. *Journal of Reading Behavior, 22*(2), 181–199.

Appendix

Excerpt from a test of passage comprehension by means of the sentence verification technique

CROWS

Of all the birds, people believe that the crow is the biggest pest. He is a large black bird with strong wings and a tough bill that can be put to many uses. He eats all kinds of food, such as fruits, seeds, grains, birds' eggs, and garbage. Being such a hardy eater, he has no trouble finding food even in the winter. Crows rise early in the morning to look for food. They go about in large flocks. They talk noisily to each other. When they arrive in an area to feed, they scare away other birds. They raid farmers' crops and even hens' nests in the barnyard. Men have tried to scare crows away from their fields. And they have tried to keep them from taking over the land. But they have not been able to keep these clever birds from causing trouble.

Read each sentence carefully. Is the idea of the sentence found in the passage? If it is, circle YES. If it is not, circle NO.

YES   NO   1. Crows fly from place to place in big groups. (Paraphrase)
YES   NO   2. Of all the birds, people believe that the crow is the biggest pest. (Original)
YES   NO   3. Crows rise late in the morning to look for food. (Meaning change)
YES   NO   4. Young crows learn to fly when they are about four weeks old. (Distractor)

Assessment of word-finding disorders in children and adolescents

Lynn S. Snyder, PhD, CCC-SLP
Professor
Department of Communicative Disorders
California State University, Long Beach
Long Beach, California

Dawn Godley, MA
Speech Pathology Clinical Services
Providence Speech and Hearing Center
Orange, California

AT ONE TIME OR ANOTHER, every normal speaker* experiences difficulty in finding or retrieving words. Indeed, word finding appears to be a language ability that is vulnerable to disruption (Goodglass, Kaplan, Weintraub, & Ackerman, 1976). Difficulty with word retrieval appears to be a ubiquitous symptom that can be related to many factors. Normal speakers may find it difficult to retrieve words when they are stressed or fatigued, or when their attention becomes divided in the presence of competing stimuli. More significantly, difficulty with word retrieval can also be symptomatic of a significant language disorder. Adults who have experienced a stroke often demonstrate initial symptoms of word-finding problems regardless of the site of the lesion or the severity of the insult (Goodglass, 1980). For some stroke patients, the symptom is fleeting. In others it persists, characterizing their acquired language disorder.

---

*For ease of language, terms such as normal speakers, normal adults, and normal children will be used to denote persons with normal language acquisition.

Top Lang Disord, 1992,13(1),15–32
© 1992 Aspen Publishers, Inc.

Similarly, almost all normal children and adolescents experience difficulty finding words at one time or another. This often occurs under conditions similar to those observed for adult speakers. In addition, a number of language-disordered and learning-disabled children and adolescents manifest this symptom with varying degrees of severity and under a wide variety of conditions (Schwartz & Solot, 1980). Often, the word-finding deficits observed in language-disordered and learning-disabled children and adolescents do not seem to be as severe as those evidenced in adult stroke patients. This lack of severity, the heterogeneity of the pediatric samples studied, and the variability observed in children's word-finding behaviors sometimes can make the differential diagnosis of word-finding deficits in children problematic. Further, the source of children's word-finding problems seems to vary. Researchers have found it difficult to disentangle the influence of storage elaboration, phonological encoding in memory, and temporal resolution factors.

Words are the very "stuff" of which language is made. Consequently, word-finding deficits can significantly compromise a child's ability not only to communicate but also to acquire those academic skills that involve the retrieval of words from the lexicon (Wallach & Butler, 1984). Thus it is crucial to identify and address this specific aspect of child language disorders.

WORD-FINDING DEFICITS AND THEIR IMPACT

A child or adolescent's *word-finding deficit* has been defined as a problem in generating the specific word that any given situation, stimulus, or sentence context evokes (Rapin & Wilson, 1978). The symptoms of such a deficit have been described in the clinical literature as including frequent pauses, repetitions, circumlocutionary behaviors, production of fillers, and those nonverbal phonetic comments described in the sociolinguistic literature (Dittmann, 1972) as back-channel responses (e.g., "uhmm, err"), as well as nonspecific words (e.g., "thing" and "stuff") (Wiig & Semel, 1983). Often, the expressive language of children experiencing word-retrieval problems, such as some groups of learning-disabled children, has been described as inarticulate despite few frank syntactic formulation errors. Considering the type of linguistic and paralinguistic compensatory behaviors adopted by these youngsters (e.g., use of back-channel responses, nonspecific terms, and fillers), it is not surprising that their listeners perceive them in this way. Such behaviors make effective communication difficult. The imprecise messages produced by children and adolescents with word-finding deficits leave listeners confused or uncertain when there is not sufficient contextual support from the preceding conversational turns or from the surrounding environment to clarify the message.

Over the years, word-finding deficits have also been associated with reading disabilities. Researchers have suggested that fast and accurate word retrieval is a skill that may be related to reading in specific ways. (See Just & Carpenter, 1987, and Kamhi & Catts, 1989, for reviews.) Naming and reading are thought to be complex, interactive processes occurring at different levels of processing and require the individual to handle semantic as well as phonological information (Wolf,

1984). The precise nature of the relationship and similarity of the lexical access required for the tasks of naming and reading has been widely discussed and has motivated many theoretical frameworks (Gordon, 1983; Marslen-Wilson, 1989). (See Wolf and Segal in this issue for further discussion on this subject.)

Researchers have noted often that support for some type of relationship between naming and reading may be found in the observation that many poor readers perform significantly worse than normally achieving readers on naming tasks (Catts, 1989; Lovett, 1984; Wolf, 1986). Some researchers have suggested that depressed word-finding skills may influence a reader's ability to retrieve the verbal label to which the printed word is related. For example, Cicci (1980) and Rubin and Liberman (1983) have noted parallels between the oral and written language behaviors of children, suggesting that the relationship between word-finding deficits and poor lexical access in reading may be more than correlational. Other researchers have viewed the relationship as predictive-—that is, one in which poor naming skills observed at early grade levels are seen as predictive of later reading problems (Walsh, Price, & Gillingham, 1988). Recently, researchers have drawn attention to similarities in the subprocesses evoked during reading and naming, suggesting that an underlying processing or representational deficit may be responsible for the correlation (Wolf, 1991).

Regardless of the nature or loci of the hypothesized relationships, the clinical reality remains that word-finding deficits have been documented in many reading-disabled youngsters (Snyder & Downey, 1991), as well as in children with more generalized oral language impairment (Leonard, 1988), and that a number of the reading-disabled children sustain significant word-finding deficits over time (Snyder & Downey, 1991; Wolff, Michel, & Ovrut, 1990). Thus there seems to be a significant proportion of school children and adolescents with word-finding deficits whose needs must be addressed.

PSYCHOLINGUISTIC CONSIDERATIONS IN NAMING

Speech and language evaluations for children with suspected word-finding deficits should include the systematic assessment of naming. Such assessments are often limited by how comparatively little we know about the development of word retrieval as compared with other components of language processing and production. As a result, most diagnostic assessments have been motivated by the theories and findings from research conducted on adults, modified in light of the relatively few developmental findings available. Our ability to assess word finding successfully in children may be compromised by researchers' failure to study children's naming during the school years from a developmental perspective or in a manner that relates naming to robust developmental phenomena (e.g., to Piagetian views and milestones of conceptual development or to the developmental elaboration of concepts).

The literature on studies with adults is replete with theories of lexical access. (See Gordon, 1983, and Marslen-Wilson, 1989, for reviews.) The theoretical frameworks and their supporting investigations are rather explicit in nature. Given the specificity of these frameworks and our less well-developed notions of the developmental factors involved in naming, it would be difficult to adopt any one framework and endorse it as a way of conceptualizing children's word-finding problems without the requisite developmental research. Until such data are available, one way to think about word finding, and word-finding deficits in particular, might be to examine the factors that influence word finding in normal adults and determine whether there is evidence that these factors affect word finding in normal children in a similar manner. In addition, other documented evidence of variables that seem to disrupt children's word-finding performance needs to be considered. This information can then be used to evaluate the informal and formal standardized measures presently available to practicing clinicians.

Wolf (1984) has pointed out that the variables that influence fast and accurate word retrieval seem to fall into two general categories: those intrinsic to the stimulus (e.g., word frequency) and those extrinsic to the stimulus (e.g., the task demand). In addition, the integrity of the individual's linguistic, cognitive, and oral motor systems plays an obvious key role in successful performance on naming tasks.

Intrinsic variables that influence word retrieval

If words are examined to determine what makes them easier or more difficult for normal adults to retrieve, several findings can be reported from the literature on this population. First, the *frequency* with which the word occurs significantly affects ease of naming (Oldfield & Wingfield, 1965). The more frequently a word occurs, the more easily it is retrieved. Conversely, the less frequently it occurs, the greater

difficulty the speaker will have in retrieval. The effect of frequency is similarly observed in children's naming (Leonard, Nippold, Kail, & Hale, 1983; Milianti & Cullinan, 1974). Frequency is often considered the strong correlate of *familiarity,* so that the words that occur most frequently are thought to be the most familiar. *Age of acquisition* is also thought to influence ease of retrieval (Carroll & White, 1973). In other words, the earlier the word is acquired by the individual, the easier it is to retrieve it.

In addition, the *category type* to which a word belongs may also influence its retrieval. Words from prototypic categories such as fruits or vegetables are more easily retrieved than words from well-defined categories such as months of the year for which there is a small set of semantic features needed for the selection of members (Armstrong, Gleitman, & Gleitman, 1983). Further, the *degree of abstractness* of the word can influence its retrieval. It has been well documented that concrete words are more easily named than abstract words (Stowe, 1988). It might be argued, however, that many of these variables may overlap. Are not high-frequency, familiar words acquired early in life, and do they not often represent more concrete and prototypic categories? Results of studies of the composition of normal children's initial lexicons (Bretherton & Bates, 1984; Snyder, Bates, & Bretherton, 1981) support such a contention.

Fried-Oken's report (1984) on the development of fast and accurate naming in a sample of normal children supports the notion that frequency and concreteness affect children's ability to name. Further, her findings indicated that, as children mature, they find it easier to name more abstract and less frequently occurring words. In addition, she found that there was a hierarchy of difficulty for *word class*. Children found it easier to name concrete nouns than to name verbs, adjectives, and abstract nouns.

Extrinsic variables that influence word retrieval

Results of most of the studies conducted with adults indicate that the *context* in which word retrieval occurs significantly influences adults' ability to retrieve words quickly and accurately. Research findings suggest that naming in the context of a sentence completion frame is easier for normal adults than is confrontation naming (i.e., naming a pictured object) and that word retrieval in both of these contexts is easier than naming to definition (Myers-Pease & Goodglass, 1978). Rudel, Denckla, Broman, and Hirsch (1980) replicated this effect for children. In addition, the *syntactic requirements* of the task also seem to affect naming in both children and adults (Wolf, 1984). The more difficult the sentence to be formulated, the fewer resources that the adult or child will have available for word retrieval since the formulation requirements may use an inordinate share of the available resources (Snyder & Becker, 1981).

Although the *cognitive operativity of the input* has not been reported to make a difference in the speed and accuracy of word retrieval in normal adults, it does seem to have a significant effect on children (Rudel et al., 1980). Rudel et al. (1980) noted that in their sample children younger than 6 years performed more accurately when objects were used. Further, when children and adults are asked to name words rapidly in a way that requires *continuous naming*, their performance is worse than in discrete naming (Katz & Shankweiler, 1985; Stanovich, Feeman, & Cunningham, 1983). Such contexts are composed of a series of line drawings presented in a row. Subjects are then asked to name each item in the series as rapidly as possible. Such rapid automatized naming (or RAN) tasks have been used widely in studies with children because they seem to discriminate between good and poor readers (Wolf, 1984).

Reports in the literature on word finding in adults have made it clear that word retrieval is easier in some contexts than in others. The major factor that seems to facilitate word finding in adults is the effect of priming. *Priming* refers to the effect of a preceding word or words on the individual's ability to retrieve or recall a target word. Long a hallmark of the literature on memory (Glass & Holyoak, 1986), priming seems to have a strong and pervasive effect of all types of lexical access (Balota & Duchek, 1989), including naming. The more closely associated the prime is to the target word, the faster the target word is retrieved (Balota & Duchek, 1989). Further, the use of superordinate category primes or cues facilitates naming in normal and aphasic adults (Becker-Caplan, 1991). Results of studies conducted by Ceci (1983) and Kail, Hale, Leonard, and Nippold (1984) suggest that school-aged children likewise profit from category primes or cues. Similarly, results of studies conducted with the use of the Boston Naming Test (Kaplan, Goodglass, & Weintraub, 1983) on samples of children suggest that categorical primes may help older children.

Thus, information in the literature seems to indicate that intrinsic variables such as the frequency, familiarity, degree of abstractness, category type, age of acquisition, and class of the target word influence the ease of its retrieval in both normal adults and children. Similarly, variables extrinsic to the words themselves, such as the context of the task, its syntactic requirements, discrete versus continuous instances of naming, and the presence of primes, also have a significant impact on the ease of word finding in children and adults. Consequently, clinical consideration of these variables would seem to be crucial to the assessment of word finding in language-disordered children and adolescents, the selection of clinical instruments, and the interpretation of children's performance during direct assessment and observation. Another important consideration in these latter instances would be the very nature of the responses of the language-disordered child.

Behaviors indicative of word-finding difficulty

The factors that influence fast and accurate word retrieval in adults and children also elicit notable error-related behaviors. These behaviors include the nature of target word substitutions, extended response times, reduced accuracy, and performance trade-offs.

Word substitution behaviors

When adults and children experience difficulty in finding words, they often produce erroneous words as substitutions for the target words. Certain characteristics of these substitutions are particularly noteworthy. When adults make errors, they may produce words that are *semantically related*—that is, words in the same seman-

tic category such as "dog" for "cat." Similarly, normally developing children engaged in confrontation-naming tasks make this type of error most of the time (Fried-Oken, 1984). Adults may also produce words that are *phonologically related*—that is, words whose phonetic shape is similar to the target words such as "goose dryer" for "screwdriver" (Fay & Cutler, 1977). In addition, children may make errors in interpreting the visual stimulus, or *perceptual errors* (Fried-Oken, 1984) (e.g., misperceiving a cashew as a crescent moon), a behavior that has been reported for aphasic (Caramazza, Berndt, & Brownell, 1982) but not normal adults. When these perceptual errors are observed in children's word-finding performance, they are more likely instances of misperceptions of the visual stimulus than retrieval errors.

Of particular note is the phenomenon that both normal adults and normal children older than 8 years generally produce error words that are from the *same grammatical class* as the target word (Fried-Oken, 1984; Weigel-Crump & Dennis, 1986). Younger children, however, have been observed producing words that are *syntagmatically* or *sequentially related.* That is, when the target word is "dog," they may produce the word "barks" or "runs." Substitution errors of this type are thought to reflect the early organization of children's lexicons, which may be less categorically driven before the age of 7 years. Thus it appears that the word-substitution errors produced by children when they are searching for a specified target word are not random. Rather, they seem to reflect the organization of the lexicon into semantic categories. Further, Balota (in press) suggests that the preservation of grammatical class observed here may indicate the influence of interactive processing.

Performance characteristics

In addition to the verbal behaviors that are indicative of word-finding difficulty, other behavioral responses may suggest word-finding problems—namely, the accuracy and speed of the response itself. Most studies on word finding in both children and adults have been designed to judge subjects' responses in terms of the speed and accuracy of each response, given findings from the fields of cognitive psychology and psycholinguistics. (See German, 1989; Leonard, 1988; and Stanovich, 1990, for reviews.) These data suggest that the reaction time or response latency as well as accuracy can indicate the subjects' ease of processing the information. *Reaction time* or *response latency* refers to the duration of time from the moment that the subject is shown an item to the time that he or she begins the response. Shorter response latencies are thought to reflect greater ease of processing the specific item or greater skill on the part of the subject. Following this reasoning, easier items should be named faster and more difficult ones should take more time for normal children to name. *Accuracy* refers to whether the target word is retrieved correctly on the first response. (See also Nippold in this issue.)

A final observation regarding word finding in normal children indicates that their word retrieval under the stress of a speeded response is characterized by the effect of *performance trade-offs* that occur in other areas of human motor responses. Given a request for speed and accuracy of response, children who find rapid naming

difficult appear to adopt a time–accuracy trade-off response bias, which will allow them to respond to at least one of the requested conditions, speed or accuracy. Consequently, they may trade speed for accuracy, naming many items quickly but making a large number of errors. Or, they may choose to name items very slowly but very accurately. If they find word retrieval particularly difficult, they may not be able to compensate for any relative weaknesses, naming both slowly and making many errors. On the other hand, those children who find rapid naming an easy task tend to name both quickly and accurately. Thus response biases that are based on the resources that the child has available to complete the task may also influence the nature of the child's naming responses.

It is clear that many factors need to be considered in the assessment of word finding in children. Those informal and formal standardized measures that take these variables into consideration when evaluating children's responses would appear to be the measures of choice. With this in mind, measures of word finding are discussed later with the use of the framework of the psycholinguistic considerations that have been developed here.

Information on any individual child's word finding can come from many sources. Clinicians can obtain relevant information from collaborative referral, classroom observations, and the systematic assessment of word finding in different contexts.

SCREENING FOR WORD-FINDING DISORDERS IN THE CLASSROOM

In recent years, the provision of speech and language services in educational settings has changed dramatically. The role of the speech-language pathologist as a collaborator with or consultant to the classroom teacher has expanded (Silliman & Wilkinson, 1991). Initial attempts to screen for or to identify children and adolescents with word-retrieval deficits are ideally suited to begin in this context. Providing classroom teachers with inservice education and referral forms that describe characteristics of significant word-finding deficits is helpful in beginning the identification. Teacher observation forms focused exclusively on word retrieval (German, 1992) or those that include items addressing word finding allow clinicians to optimize their time. In addition, any inservice instruction provided to classroom teachers will help increase the reliability of their use of observational checklists (Secord & Wiig, 1990).

Neither checklists nor inservice education can substitute for classroom observation of the students about whom teachers are concerned. Classroom observation allows the clinician to determine whether the student's observed difficulties with word retrieval occurred with known vocabulary in familiar contexts across situations or whether they were situationally driven—that is, elicited by the need to produce unfamiliar, less frequently used vocabulary or unfamiliar discourse topics. Similarly, it allows the clinician to observe whether the student's problems were culturally driven, by either nonnative fluency in English or cultural differences that may constrain the speaker's responses (Westby, 1991). Difficulty in finding words that are familiar vocabulary items has been observed to be differentially diagnostic of children considered to have clinically significant word-finding deficits (German, 1982). These observations, along with sub-

sequent consultation with the classroom teacher, can then be used to determine which students will need referral for speech and language evaluations.

DIRECT ASSESSMENT OF WORD FINDING DURING EVALUATIONS

School-aged children and adolescents with suspected word-finding disorders who have been referred for speech and language evaluations may be treated in two ways: direct assessment with diagnostic instruments and clinical observation of their performance during spontaneous conversation. The prevailing clinical bias in the discipline of communication disorders has been to make use of both methods when working with youngsters from the mainstream culture. Snyder and Becker (1981) have cautioned against the solitary use of informal clinical observation to gather information on which a diagnostic impression of word-finding disorder will be formulated. Children's word retrieval during spontaneous discourse may be influenced negatively by factors such as topic familiarity (cited earlier).

The identification of word-finding deficits that are related to underlying cognitive and linguistic-processing deficits and are not situationally artifactual (e.g., related to less familiar discourse topics and the associated vocabulary or cultural differences) rests on baseline information about the child's receptive vocabulary skills, as well as on the determination that the child comprehends the target words to be presented in the naming tasks. If the child's comprehension of the target words cannot be determined, the clinician cannot rule out that the child's difficulty with the word is related to receptive language factors.

Hence, it seems important that the assessment of word finding in children makes some provision for this factor.

There are two general types of instruments that have been used for the direct assessment of word retrieval in children: informal or experimental measures and formal standardized measures. The informal or experimental instruments have been used primarily for research purposes and standardized tests which are available for more general use. Most of these instruments sample children's word finding in the single word context; one recently developed standardized instrument samples word retrieval during discourse.

Informal or experimental measures

Researchers from the fields of communicative disorders, reading disabilities, and adult aphasia have developed a number of informal or experimental tools for the assessment of word finding. Although these measures were developed primarily for experimental studies, some have been used clinically to assess children's word-finding difficulties. This is feasible when the child meets all of the subject selection criteria (e.g., age, gender, socioeconomic status, ethnicity, and cognitive level), excluding language and reading level, as the normal sample in the study. In such instances, these measures can provide useful information.

The following discussion will focus on those measures referenced most frequently in the literature—namely, the Northwestern Word Latency Test (Rutherford & Tesler, 1971), the Word Naming Test (Weigel-Crump & Dennis, 1986), the Rapid Automatized Naming (RAN) (Denckla & Rudel, 1974, 1976), the Rapid Alternating Stimulus Test (RAS) (Wolf,

1984, 1986), the Boston Naming Test (Kaplan, Goodglass, & Weintraub, 1983), and the Controlled Word Association Test or "FAS" Set Test (Benton, 1973). Typically, most of these word-finding measures have provided information on children's ability to retrieve single words in picture-naming contexts. They include tasks that assess discrete or continuous naming with one measure assessing associative naming. With the exception of the Boston Naming Test, which contains provisional norms for children, and the Word Latency Test, these informal or experimental measures lack normative data. Few of these measures have been subjected to studies of their reliability, validity, and internal consistency.

Northwestern Word Latency Test

The Northwestern Word Latency Test (Rutherford & Telser, 1971) was designed to differentiate dysfluent children from children with word-finding difficulties. Response time was the index of skilled performance, and target word comprehension was controlled as items not known were eliminated from the assessment. Little attempt was made by these authors, however, to control systematically for psycholinguistic characteristics of the stimuli (e.g., word frequency, abstractness, imagery).

Word Naming Test

The Word Naming Test (Weigel-Crump & Dennis, 1986) was developed to identify word-retrieval deficits in language-disordered children with documented brain injury. Children are asked to name visually and verbally presented stimuli, including definitions and rhyming cues. Open-ended definitions, organized according to semantic attributes, are presented one at a time.

This measure also contains a set of stimuli in which the child produces a name in a designated hierarchical category (e.g., animal) that rhymes with a pseudoword cue presented by the examiner (e.g., "Can you tell me an animal that rhymes with 'gat'?"), as well as a set of pictorial stimuli for the child to name. Provisions are also made for recording speed and accuracy as well as analyzing errors. Further, the stimuli are controlled for word frequency, imagery, concreteness, meaningfulness, number of attributes, pleasantness, associate cue values, and familiarity.

Although the nouns presented are all known to be acquired by age 4 years, the measure does not explicitly control for each child's comprehension of the items, nor does it provide for priming effects. More importantly, it assumes that the child has developed sufficient metalinguistic skills to permit rhyming cues to be facilitative in retrieving the word. This assumption is certainly invalid for a great majority of reading-disabled and language-impaired children for whom the development of metalinguistic skills is significantly delayed (Catts, 1989).

RAN and RAS

Two measures have emerged from the literature on reading disabilities—the RAN (Denckla & Rudel, 1976) and the RAS (Wolf, 1986). These measures, used to differentiate the word-finding skills of children with and without reading disabilities, examine children's serial naming speed for pictured familiar and known objects, colors, digits, and letters. (See Wolf and Segal in this issue for a discussion.)

The RAN and RAS naming tasks differ in that the RAS presents the naming stimuli from different semantic categories alternately (e.g., letter–number–letter–number). The accuracy of the subjects' responses, as well as the total time that it takes to finish naming the series, is recorded.

The RAN and RAS allow the clinician to observe the speed of a child's responses. Since older children have been described to ceiling out for accuracy on these measures, the opportunity to observe speed–accuracy trade-offs on these measures has been limited. The measures cited, however, do not report the use of systematic controls for the effects of word frequency, familiarity, and age of acquisition. One set of RAN stimuli, developed by Wolf (1984) for use in addition to three of Denckla and Rudel's original sets, did control for word frequency, phonological difficulty, and developmental influences on semantic sets. Further, although it is possible for clinicians to analyze a child's errors, these measures have not made any systematic provision for the categorization of errors.

Boston Naming Test and Controlled Word Association (or FAS Set) Test

From the literature on adult aphasia, two measures have emerged. One has been used frequently with children and contains provisional norms for the school-aged population. The other has been reported in neuropsychological studies of reading-disabled children.

The first instrument, the Boston Naming Test, involves the child or adult in confrontation naming. *Confrontation naming* involves presenting stimuli one at a time and asking the individual to name each stimulus. This measure records the accuracy of the subject's responses, but does not take into account response time.

Experimental measures of this type may under-identify older children with word-retrieval deficits because reaction times appear to be more sensitive measures of word retrieval in older children (Snyder & Downey, 1991). On the other hand, the items on this measure have been controlled for factors such as word frequency and phonological difficulty from the adult, but not the developmental, perspective. Thus, some of the vocabulary items (e.g., *asparagus* and *canoe*) are less likely to be familiar to children.

Further, the Boston Naming Test does not sample different stimulus contexts or semantic categories. Recently, Wolf (1990) developed a multiple-choice vocabulary item recognition test for the Boston Naming Test that controls for the individual's comprehension of the test items. In its commercially available form, however, the Boston Naming Test does not control for comprehension of test items. Wolf's comprehension check represents a strong addition. The Boston Naming Test does, however, provide the clinician with guidance in performing error analyses, as well as an opportunity to prime with semantic and phonetic cues and to observe the differential effect of such cuing on naming accuracy.

The second word-retrieval measure coming from the perspective of aphasiology is the Controlled Word Association (or FAS Set) Test. With this measure of verbal fluency subjects are asked to name as many words beginning with "f" in a minute. Adult norms are available on this measure, but the test depends on a knowledge of sound–letter correspondence for its execution. Obviously, any child's failure to develop sound–letter correspondence will unduly penalize the child's performance. Accuracy and time are obviously considered in this task, leaving all remaining factors unconsidered.

Formal standardized measures

Among the standardized assessment instruments available to clinicians, three are designed specifically to assess word-finding skills in children and adolescents. In addition, one multicomponent test battery and its recent revision contain subtests that focus on word retrieval per se. Prominent among the standardized measures of word retrieval are German's Test of Word Finding (TWF) (1986/1989), Test of Adolescent/Adult Word Finding (TAWF) (1990b), and Test of Word Finding in Discourse (TWFD) (1991).

TWF and TAWF

The TWF (German, 1986/1989) and the TAWF (German, 1990) focus on the systematic assessment of children's naming skills in a variety of contexts: confrontation naming for different word classes and categories, sentence completion naming, and naming to description. Both instruments check target word comprehension of all naming errors. In addition, both measures take into account the factors of word frequency, familiarity, category type, word class, hierarchy of difficulty, response time, and accuracy, as well as error analysis. The only factor that is not controlled is the observation of priming effects on a child's word retrieval. On the whole, these measures seem to provide a comprehensive assessment of word finding in children and adolescents. This strength, however, may limit their use in instances in which the clinician does not have sufficient time available to administer the tests.

TWFD

The TWFD German's (1991) latest measure, assesses children's word retrieval during discourse-production tasks. It presents pictorial stimuli to a child to elicit a narrative language sample. The sample is then analyzed with respect to *productivity*—the total number of words and t-units in the narrative—and *incidence of word-finding behaviors*—the percentage of t-units containing one or more of the following word-finding behaviors: repetitions, reformulations, substitutions, insertions, empty words, time fillers, and delays. The normative data indicate that children whose narratives contain a high proportion (33%) of t-units containing one or more word-finding behaviors can be regarded as manifesting word-finding difficulties on the TWFD.

Although the primary index of the TWFD is the incidence of word-finding behaviors in narratives, formulation of hypotheses regarding children's word-finding skills are recommended on the basis of the productivity index. German (1991) cautions, however, that low-productivity scores do not always mean that a child has word-finding problems because factors other than retrieval skills can contribute to low productivity in discourse. Concerns about competition for resources (Snyder & Downey, 1984), in particular the effect of topic familiarity on resources available for discourse (Anderson, Spiro, & Anderson, 1978; Goetz & Armbruster, 1980), suggest that clinicians should interpret positive findings on the TWFD with caution. That

is, the production of narrative discourse not only involves the retrieval of words, but also includes the organization of the components of narrative discourse. It is well known that children produce less well-formed narratives for topics with which they are less familiar or which are elicited in less familiar situational contexts. Lack of familiarity with a discourse topic or discourse context may require the allocation of a larger share of the available resources, leaving the child with insufficient resources available for word retrieval or the formulation of sentences. Those children with formulation deficits would suffer similar limitations on their resources. The TWFD, however, should identify these children at the outset. These youngsters would most likely score significantly below the norms on the t-unit metric from this assessment. In fact, the TWFD manual cautions against applying the TWFD norms to narratives of less than 21 t-units. In these cases, the clinician would then reserve the possibility of a word-finding deficit and consider the rival explanation that children's word-finding behaviors might be possible evidence of the reduced resources available to the child given the greater demand placed on them for formulation. German (1991) has recommended additional language assessment, home reports, and classroom observation for these children to clarify better the nature of their low-productivity problems in discourse.

Interactionist accounts of lexical acquisition stress the notion that vocabulary acquisition is embedded in event contexts (Chapman, in press). This embedding, then, results in the encapsulation of more recently acquired lexical entries before the decontextualization that takes place over time (Bates, Bretherton, & Snyder, 1988; Snyder et al., 1981). The assessment of word finding in discourse can prove difficult because the event, topic, or theme being narrated may be one that is not well elaborated in the child's system or one so recently acquired that the associated lexical items are not sufficiently decontextualized.

Current thinking and German's own remarks to clinicians suggest that this measure may be used best as part of a larger testing battery in which these other structural components of language are assessed. Additional testing would also clarify the presence of formulation problems.

In conclusion, the TWFD also makes a logical addition to any test battery in which the TWF has been administered, allowing the clinician to observe the child's word finding not only in single word naming but in discourse as well.

Clinical Evaluation of Language Functions (CELF) and Clinical Evaluation of Language Fundamentals-Revised (CELF-R)

Some multimeasure tests contain subtests directed to the assessment of word finding in different contexts. The early version of the CELF (Wiig & Semel, 1983) contained two subtests that directly used naming: Producing Words on Confrontation and Producing Word Associations. The first subtest was essentially a RAN procedure in which children were asked to name as rapidly as possible colored geometric shapes presented in rows on a page. In this measure both accuracy and the total time taken to complete the measure are recorded. In the latter subtest, a version of the classic neuropsychological "animal set test" (Lezak, 1976), children are asked to name as many animals as possible in one minute. This subtest examines word retrieval within a specific category. By using words and categories with a high degree of frequency, these subtests do control for some of the psycholinguistic factors that affect word retrieval. Since highly familiar and frequently used words and categories from the mainstream culture were used, however, clinicians often reported ceiling effects for accuracy, especially on the confrontation naming task, as acknowledged by the authors of its revision (Semel, Wiig, & Secord, 1987). For this reason it was dropped from the revised assessment.

In its revised form (Semel et al., 1987), the CELF-R contains a modification of the Word Associations subtest that includes more abstract categories. Thus, this verbal fluency subtest may be better able to discriminate children with deficient word retrieval within categories. Although this subtest offers information regarding only one dimension of children's word finding, it does explore a word-retrieval task that historically has been considered a robust index of individual differences when taken into consideration with other assessment data (Horn, 1985; Lezak, 1976).

In summary, a number of informal or experimental and standardized formal measures of word finding are currently available to clinicians. In light of the central role of word finding in language production, it is crucial that it should be included in assessment. The accurate characterization of any child's language should consider all aspects of language comprehension and production, particularly those with which the child has demonstrated difficulty.

INDIVIDUAL DIFFERENCES AND NAMING

Whether one holds to a modular or an interactionist view of language processing and production, any assessment of a child or adolescent suspected of having word-finding deficits should be comprehensive. It should take into consideration the child's existing diagnostic profile of other language processing and production strengths and weaknesses, history of language learning, and existing lexical skills.

Existing diagnostic profile

Assessment of the child with suspected word-finding problems should consider his or her other language and information processing strengths and weaknesses. The child's comprehension and production of syntactic and morphological structures, phonological repertoire, vocabulary comprehension, and discourse processing and production should be examined, in addition to his or her naming skills. Of particular importance is the child's vocabulary comprehension. It would be difficult to expect children with impoverished lexicons (i.e., with limited comprehension as well as expression entries) to engage in fluent word retrieval during nonformulaic speech beyond the level of their comprehension skills. Further, since naming depends on the child's ability to articulate on demand, it should also consider the structure and functioning of his or her oral peripheral musculature. A less efficient oral-motor mechanism may make greater demands during the word-retrieval pro-

cess than originally anticipated (Huttenlocher, 1984). Thus other weaknesses within the child's language system may demand more resources at a point in processing or production, which does not leave sufficient resources in the pool for rapid and accurate word retrieval.

Individual differences

Another consideration that may be relevant to the assessment of word-retrieval deficits in children and adolescents is the child's expressive language style. Some youngsters may be at greater risk for word-retrieval deficits, given their habitual style of expressive language along the continuum of formulaic to referential speech (Bates et al., 1988). Or, it may be that children with language disorders in general are, by definition, more formulaic in their expressive language (Bates & Thal, 1991). That is, they may make greater use of clichés, highly routinized expressions, pronouns, and so forth, in their expressive language. Reasoning in the opposite direction, their style may be indicative of difficulty in retrieving specific vocabulary items. In either case, the more a child or adolescent relies on formulaic phrases, clichés, and the like, the less frequently the youngster may engage in the retrieval of specific words.

Because practice tends to make items more automatic, children who produce fewer names may, in some sense, reduce their own opportunities for engaging in word retrieval. In fact, their expressive style may contribute to continued difficulty with word retrieval. It is important, then, to consider many different factors, especially other verbal skills, when assessing word retrieval deficits.

WORD-RETRIEVAL DEMANDS IN OTHER ASSESSMENT CONTEXTS

Many language and cognitive assessments rely on a youngster's verbal responses. In some instances, the production of a specified word or words is required for the child or adolescent to be credited with a correct answer to a test item. In such instances, a word-retrieval deficit could have a serious impact on the child's performance.

Two popular measures that have been designed to assess expressive vocabulary are the Expressive One-Word Picture Vocabulary-Revised (Gardner, 1991), which is used with children aged 2 through 11 years, and the Expressive One-Word Picture Vocabulary: Upper Extension (Gardner, 1990), which is used with adolescents aged 12 through 15 years. These tests actually involve some confrontation naming. The child is shown a line drawing and asked to name it. The test scoring focuses on accuracy. Although these measures have been designed to assess expressive vocabulary, children with significant word-retrieval deficits may perform poorly on them.

Similarly, measures that contain tasks or subtests in which the child is required to name a synonym or an antonym for a specified word—for example, the Synonyms and Antonyms subtests from the Word Test (Barrett, Huisingh, Zachman, & Jorgensen, 1980) and the Word Opposites subtest of the Detroit Tests of Learning Aptitude-3 (Hammill, 1991)—may be problematic for the child with word-retrieval deficits. Fortunately, clinicians who are well trained in task analysis can recognize the impact of the child's word-retrieval deficit on his or her performance

on these measures of language and information processing.

Another serious concern is the youngster's performance on cognitive measures in which deficient performance (i.e., failure to produce a specified word) may be interpreted as an indication of or contributing to significant conceptual or cognitive deficit. Clinicians have been aware for some time of the demands that the Stanford-Binet Intelligence Scale (Terman & Merrill, 1973) and the Slossen Intelligence Test for Children and Adults (Slossen, 1977) place on youngsters' word-retrieval skills. For example, the Picture Vocabulary, Naming Objects, Opposite Analogies, Rhymes, and Word Naming components of the Stanford-Binet explicitly require word-retrieval responses from children. Similarly, the Slossen Intelligence Test contains items at the older age levels that require word retrieval.

Reasoning in this same direction, the Magic Window, Expressive Vocabulary, Gestalt Closure, and Faces and Places subtests of the Kaufman Assessment Battery for Children (K-ABC) (Kaufman & Kaufman, 1983) rely heavily on a child's word-retrieval skills (German, 1983). These represent one-fourth of the subtests on this measure; thus the impact of a child's word-retrieval deficit would be significant. In this same vein, the Picture Vocabulary and the Antonyms–Synonyms subtests from the earlier version of the Woodcock-Johnson Psycho-Educational Battery's (Woodcock & Johnson, 1977) Tests of Cognitive Ability rely on word-retrieval skills. Likewise, the Picture Vocabulary and the Oral Vocabulary subtests from the recent revision, the Tests of Cognitive Ability (Woodcock & Johnson, 1989), are structured in the same way. Therefore it seems there are potentially many instances in which children and adolescents with word-retrieval deficits could be unduly penalized by their language disorder on cognitive assessments. It is important, therefore, to identify youngsters' word-retrieval deficits, in addition to deficits in other language processes, and to consider the potential effects of these deficits on their performance on language and cognitive assessments.

• • •

One would think that naming objects, actions, and conditions is a relatively simple and straightforward process and that the assessment of this verbal skill would be similarly direct. The complexity of language production, however, is such that even a task so apparently simple as

naming can be influenced by many factors both internal and external to the speaker. More importantly, the surface simplicity of the task and the process is deceptive; it masks the crucial role played by word retrieval in the communicative process. The very substance of the message can be compromised seriously by word-finding disorders. Thus it is important that children and adolescents with suspected word-finding deficits be assessed in a comprehensive and systematic manner. In addition, the application of a motivated set of psycholinguistic considerations to the selection of assessment tools and the interpretation of children's word-finding behaviors on these measures and in more naturalistic contexts can only improve the accuracy of clinical judgments made and help clinicians identify the most appropriate contexts and modalities for intervention.

REFERENCES

Anderson, R., Spiro, R., & Anderson, M.C. (1978). Schemata as scaffolding for the representation of information in connected discourse. *American Educational Research Journal, 15*, 433–440.

Armstrong, S.L., Gleitman, L., & Gleitman, H. (1983). What some concepts might not be. *Cognition, 13*, 263–308.

Balota, D.A. (in press). The role of meaning in word recognition. In D.A. Balota, G.B. Flores d'Arcais, & K. Rayner (Eds.), *Comprehension processes in reading.* Hillsdale, NJ: Erlbaum.

Balota, D.A., & Duchek, J. (1989). Age-related differences in lexical access, spreading activation, and simple pronunciation. *Psychology and Aging, 3*, 84–93.

Barrett, M., Huisingh, R., Zachman, L., & Jorgensen, C. (1980). *The word test.* East Moline, IL: Linguisystems.

Bates, E., Bretherton, I., & Snyder, L. (1988). *From first words to grammar: Individual differences and dissociable mechanisms.* New York, NY: Cambridge University Press.

Bates, E. and Thal, D. (1991). Associations and dissociations in language development. In Miller, J. (Ed.), *Research on child language disorders: A decade of progress* (pp. 145–168). Austin, TX: Pro-Ed.

Becker-Caplan, L. (1991). *Well-defined and prototypic categories: Evidence from aphasia.* Unpublished doctoral dissertation, University of Denver.

Benton, A.L. (1973). The measurement of aphasic disorders. In A.C. Velasquez (Ed.), *Aspectos patologicos del lengage.* Lima, Peru: Centro Neuropsicologico.

Bretherton, I., & Bates, E. (1984). The development of representation from 10 to 28 months: Differential stability of language and symbolic play. In R.N. Emde & R.H. Harmon (Eds.), *Continuities and discontinuities in development.* New York, NY: Plenum.

Caramazza, A., Berndt, R., & Brownell, H.H. (1982). The semantic deficit hypothesis: Perceptual parsing an object classification by aphasic patients. *Brain and Language, 15*, 161–189.

Carroll, J.B., & White, M. (1973). Word frequency and age of acquisition of picture-naming latency. *Quarterly Journal of Experimental Psychology, 25*, 85–95.

Catts, H. (1989). Phonological processing deficits and reading disabilities. In A.G. Kamhi & H.W. Catts (Eds.), *Reading disabilities: A developmental language perspective.* Newton, MA: Allyn & Bacon.

Ceci, S. (1983). Automatic and purposive semantic processing characteristics of normal and language/learning-disabled children. *Developmental Psychology, 19,* 427–439.

Chapman, R. (in press). Child Talk: Assumptions of a developmental process model for early language learning. In Chapman, R. (Ed.), *Processes in language acquisition.* Chicago: Mosby Yearbook, Inc.

Cicci, R. (1980). Written language disorders. *Bulletin of the Orton Society, 30,* 240–251.

Denckla, M.B., & Rudel, R. (1974). Rapid "automatized" naming of pictured objects, colors, letters, and numbers by normal children. *Cortex, 10,* 186–202.

Denckla, M.B., & Rudel, R. (1976). Naming of object drawings by dyslexic and other learning disabled children. *Brain and Language, 3,* 1–16.

Dittmann, A.T. (1972). The body movement-speech rhythm relationship as a cue to speech encoding. In A.W. Siegman & B. Pope (Eds.), *Studies in dyadic communication* (pp. 135–151). New York: Pergamon Press.

Fay, D., & Cutler, A. (1977). Malapropisms and the structure of the mental lexicon. *Linguistic Inquiry, 8,* 505–520.

Fried-Oken, M. (1984). The development of naming skills in normal and language deficient children. Unpublished doctoral dissertation, Boston University, Boston, MA.

Gardner, M. (1990). *Expressive one-word picture vocabulary: Upper extension.* San Francisco, CA: Academic Therapy Publications.

Gardner, M. (1991). *Expressive one-word picture vocabulary-revised.* San Francisco, CA: Academic Therapy Publications.

German, D. (1982). Word-finding substitutions in children with learning disabilities. *Language, Speech and Hearing in the Schools, 13,* 223–230.

German, D. (1983a). *Analysis of word finding disorders on the Kaufman assessment battery for children (K-ABC).* San Diego, CA: Grune & Stratton.

German, D. (1986/1989). *National college of education test of word finding (TWF).* Allen, TX: DLM Teaching Resources.

German, D. (1989). A diagnostic model and a test to assess word-finding skills in children. *British Journal of Disorders of Communication, 24,* 21–39.

German, D. (1990). *National College of Education Test of Adolescent/Adult Word Finding (TAWF).* Allen, TX: DLM Teaching Resources.

German, D. (1991). *Test of Word Finding in Discourse (TWFD).* Allen, TX: DLM Teaching Resources.

German, D. (1992). *Word finding referral checklist.* Riverwoods, IL: Word Finding Material, Inc.

Glass, A.L., & Holyoak, S. (1986). *Cognition* (2nd ed.). New York, NY: Random House.

Goetz, E.T., & Armbruster, B.B. (1980). Psychological correlates of text structure. In R.J. Spiro, B. Bruce, & W.F. Brewer (Eds.), *Theoretical issues in reading comprehension* (pp. 201–220). Hillsdale, NJ: Erlbaum.

Goodglass, H. (1980). Disorders of naming following brain injury. *American Scientist, 68,* 647–655.

Goodglass, H., Kaplan, E., Weintraub, S., & Ackerman, N. (1976). The "tip of the tongue" phenomenon in aphasia. *Cortex, 12,* 145–153.

Gordon, B. (1983). Lexical access and lexical decision: Mechanism of frequency sensitivity. *Journal of Verbal Learning and Verbal Behavior, 22,* 23–44.

Hammill, D. (1991). *Detroit Tests of Learning Aptitude-3.* Austin, TX: Pro-Ed.

Horn, J. (1985). Remodeling old models of intelligence. In B.B. Wolman (Ed.), *Handbook of intelligence* (pp. 267–300). New York, NY: Wiley.

Huttenlocher, J. (1984). Word recognition and word production in children. In H. Bouma & D.G. Bouwhuis (Eds.), *Attention and performance X* (pp. 447–457). Hillsdale, NJ: Erlbaum.

Just, M., & Carpenter, P. (1987). *The psychology of reading and language comprehension.* Newton, MA: Allyn & Bacon.

Kail, R., Hale, B., Leonard, L., & Nippold, M. (1984). Lexical storage and retrieval in language-impaired children. *Applied Psycholinguistics, 5,* 37–49.

Kamhi, A.G., & Catts, H.W. (Eds.). (1989). *Reading disabilities: A developmental language perspective.* Newton, MA: Allyn & Bacon.

Kaplan, E., Goodglass, H., & Weintraub, N. (1983). *The Boston Naming Test.* Philadelphia, PA: Lea & Febiger.

Katz, R.B., & Shankweiler, D. (1985). Repetitive naming and the detection of word retrieval deficits in beginning readers. *Cortex, 21,* 617–625.

Kaufman, A., & Kaufman, N. (1983). *Kaufman Assessment Battery for Children (K-ABC).* Circle Pines, MN: American Guidance Service.

Leonard, L.B. (1988). Lexical development and processing in specific language impairment. In R. Schiefelbusch & L. Lloyd (Eds.), *Perspectives in language II.* Austin, TX: Pro-Ed.

Leonard, L.B., Nippold, M., Kail, R., & Hale, B. (1983). Picture naming in language impaired children. *Journal of Speech and Hearing Research, 26,* 609–615.

Lezak, M. (1976). *Neuropsychological assessment.* New York, NY: Oxford University Press.

Lovett, M. (1984). A developmental perspective on reading dysfunction: Accuracy and rate criteria in the subtyping of dyslexic children. *Brain and Language, 22,* 67–91.

Marslen-Wilson, W. (Ed.). (1989). *Lexical representation and process.* Cambridge, MA: MIT Press.

Milianti, F., & Cullinan, W. (1974). Effects of age and word frequency on object recognition and naming in children. *Journal of Speech and Hearing Research, 17,* 373–385.

Myers-Pease, D., & Goodglass, H. (1978). The effects of cuing in picture naming aphasea. *Cortex, 14,* 178–189.

Oldfield, R.C., & Wingfield, A. (1965). Response latencies in naming objects. *Quarterly Journal of Experimental Psychology, 17,* 273–281.

Rapin, I., & Wilson, B. (1978). Children with developmental language disability: Neurological aspects and assessment. In M. Wyke (Ed.), *Developmental dysphasia* (pp. 13–41). New York, NY: Academic Press.

Rubin, H., & Liberman, I. (1983). Exploring the oral and written language errors made by language disabled children. *Annals of Dyslexia, 33,* 110–120.

Rudel, R., Denckla, M., Broman, M., & Hirsch, S. (1980). Word finding as a function of stimulus context: Children compared with aphasic adults. *Brain and Language, 10,* 111–119.

Rutherford, D., & Tesler, E. (1971). *The Word Latency Test.* Paper presented to the Association for Children and Adults with Learning Disabilities, Chicago, IL.

Schwartz, E., & Solot, C. (1980). Response patterns characteristic of verbal expressive disorders. *Language, Speech and Hearing in the Schools, 11,* 139–144.

Secord, W., & Wiig, E. (1990). *Developing a collaborative language-intervention model in the schools.* Unpublished manuscript.

Semel, E., Wiig, E., & Secord, W. (1980). *The Clinical Evaluation of Language Fundamentals.* Columbus, OH: Charles E. Merrill.

Semel, E., Wiig, E., & Secord, W. (1987). *The Clinical Evaluation of Language Fundamentals—Revised.* New York, NY: Psychological Corp.

Silliman, E., & Wilkinson, L.C. (1991). *Communicating for learning: Observation and collaboration.* Gaithersburg, MD: Aspen Publishers.

Slossen, R.L. (1977). *Slossen intelligence test for children and adults.* East Aurora, NY: Slossen Educational Publications.

Snyder, L., Bates, E., & Bretherton, I. (1981). Content and context in early lexical development. *Journal of Child Language, 8,* 565–582.

Snyder, L., & Downey, D.M. (1984). Pragmatics and information processing. *Topics in Language Disorders, 4,* 75–86.

Snyder, L.S., & Becker, L.B. (1981, November). *Lexical accessing strategies for language and learning disabled children.* Paper presented at the American–Speech–Language–Hearing Association convention, Los Angeles, CA.

Snyder, L.S., & Downey, D.M. (1991). The language-reading relationship in normal and reading-disabled children. *Journal of Speech and Hearing Research, 34,* 129–140.

Stanovich, K. (1990). Concepts in developmental theories of reading skill: Cognitive resources, automaticity and modularity. *Developmental Review, 10,* 72–100.

Stanovich, K.E., Feeman, D.J., & Cunningham, A.E. (1983). The development of the relation between letter naming speed and reading ability. *Bulletin of Psychonomic Society, 21,* 199–202.

Stowe, L. (1988). Thematic structures and sentence comprehension. In G. Carlen & M. Tanenhaus (Eds.), *Linguistic structure in language processing.* Dordrecht, The Netherlands: Reidel.

Terman, L., & Merrill, M. (1973). *Stanford-Binet Intelligence Scale, 1972 norms edition.* Boston: Houghton-Mifflin.

Wallach, G., & Butler, K. (1984). *Language learning disabilities in school age children.* Baltimore, MD: Williams & Wilkins.

Walsh, D., Price, G., & Gillingham, M. (1988). The crucial but transitory importance of letter naming. *Reading Research Quarterly, 23,* 108–122.

Weigel-Crump, C., & Dennis, M. (1986). The development of word-finding. *Brain and Language, 27,* 1–23.

Westby, C. (1991, April). *Multicultural issues in language-learning disabilities.* Paper presented at the New York State Speech–Language–Hearing Association convention, Kiamesha Lake, NY.

Wiig, E., & Semel, E. (1983). *The clinical evaluation of language functions; Second edition.* Columbus, OH: Charles E. Merrill.

Wolf, M. (1984). Naming, reading and the dyslexias: A longitudinal overview. *Annals of Dyslexia, 34,* 87–115.

Wolf, M. (1986). Rapid alternating stimulus naming in the developmental dyslexias. *Brain and Language, 27,* 360–379.

Wolf, M. (1990). *The Boston Naming Test, Children's Version: Multiple Choice Component.* Unpublished manuscript.

Wolf, M. (1991). Naming speed and reading: The contribution of the cognitive neurosciences. *Reading Research Quarterly, 26,* 123–140.

Wolff, P., Michel, G., & Ovrut, M. (1990). Rate and timing of precision of motor coordination in developmental dyslexia. *Developmental Psychology, 26,* 349–359.

Woodcock, R.W., & Johnson, M.B. (1977). *Woodcock-Johnson Psycho-Educational Battery.* Allen, TX: DLM Teaching Resources.

Woodcock, R.W., & Johnson, M.B. (1989). *Tests of Cognitive Ability.* Allen, TX: DLM Teaching Resources.

Implementing computerized language sample analysis in the public school

Jon F. Miller, PhD
Professor
Waisman Mental Retardation Research
*   Center*
Department of Communicative Disorders
University of Wisconsin-Madison
Madison, Wisconsin

Christine Freiberg, MS
Speech-Language Pathologist
Wausau School District
Wausau, Wisconsin

Mary-Beth Rolland, MS
Speech-Language Pathologist

Mary Anne Reeves, MS
Speech-Language Pathologist
Madison Metropolitan School District
Madison, Wisconsin

IN 1982, WE BEGAN A series of projects aimed at implementing computerized language sample analysis (LSA) in public schools. To date, the project has involved more than 60 speech-language pathologists working in public schools in Wisconsin. In this article, we review our progress toward the objective of making computerized LSA available to school speech-language pathologists and offer some suggestions for doing so. In addition, we discuss the ways in which the project has led us to reconceptualize not only the

This article is based on a presentation made at the American Speech-Language-Hearing Association (ASHA) annual meeting in Seattle, Washington, November 1990. The ASHA presentation and this article are the results of the efforts of the following people: Dee Boyd, Kathleen Lyngaas, Rebecca Zutter-Brose, Beth Daggett, Marianne Gill, Marianne Kellman, Colleen Lodholtz, Katherine Pierce, and Lynda Lee Ruchti from the Madison Metropolitan School District; Jim Larson, Jan M. Molaska, Mary Clare Freeman, and Kathy Bertolino from the Cooperative Educational Service Agency No. 9, Tomahawk, WI; Claire Wyhuske, University of Wisconsin-Madison; and Brent Odell, Wisconsin State Department of Public Instruction.

Top Lang Disord, 1992,12(2),69–82
© 1992 Aspen Publishers, Inc.

language performance of individual children, but our views on the nature of language impairment in school-age populations.

The first project began in the Madison Metropolitan School District (MMSD), out of frustration with the limitations of available testing methods used to identify and describe language-impaired children. The MMSD speech-language pathologists recognized that LSA offered the most efficacious method for describing disordered language performance. Yet there were significant problems impeding the implementation of LSA throughout the district. Among these problems were the lack of a consistent transcription format, the lack of a set of standard analysis routines that would cover all levels of language production performance, and the lack of a database of language measures from normally developing children that could be used to interpret data from an individual child suspected of having a language disorder. Solutions to all of these problems were necessary before LSA could be used as a clinical tool to determine which children were developing normally and which children had language impairments evidencing an exceptional educational need.

Solving these problems required substantial effort in two areas. First, standard sampling and analysis methods had to be developed using a single transcription format. This single format would provide conventions for transcribing all possible features of productive language necessary for documenting developmental delay and disordered performance. The second area of substantial effort was the development of a database of language samples from

school-aged children in relevant speaking conditions. Our progress in each of these areas has been fundamental to our progress in implementing LSA in the schools.

CREATING STANDARD ANALYSIS PROCEDURES: COMPUTER PROGRAM DEVELOPMENT

Members of the Language Analysis Laboratory at the University of Wisconsin-Madison had been at work since 1981 developing computer methods for LSA. These efforts were aimed at developing computer solutions to the tedious and time-consuming process of analyzing language samples to assess a broad range of language performance features. In the fall of 1982, we completed the first prototype of Systematic Analysis of Language Transcripts (SALT; Miller & Chapman, 1982), a computer program designed to analyze language transcripts from children and adults in a variety of speaking conditions. The success of our initial version of SALT provided insight into the ways computer programs can increase the efficiency and reduce the tedium of the analysis portion of the language sample analysis process. We also began to see how computer analysis contributed to the development of a consistent transcription format, because computer analysis requires all transcripts to be done the same way, using a standard notation system for identifying features of words and utterances.

Our first goal with the SALT program was to develop standard analysis routines covering all language levels: lexical, morphological, syntactic, semantic, and pragmatic. The first version of SALT generated a number of standard measures that investigators studying language development have used to characterize progress, including mean length of utterance, type-token ratio, total number of words, number of different words, and number of utterances per speaking turn. Subsequent versions of SALT have elaborated these metrics to include many others, and have led to the development of a second program that allows users to implement their own analyses of the transcript. This part of the SALT analysis program acknowledges the complexity of language performance, the variability of disordered language performance, and the need for human judgment about many aspects of language that would be ambiguous in completely automated computer analyses. This module of SALT was designed to support clinicians and researchers in their efforts to conduct a wide variety of language analyses motivated by the characteristics of individual subjects.

The reciprocal nature of the relationship between the development of the computerized LSA programs and the solution of various problems required for implementing computerized LSA in various clinical settings soon became evident. LSA has four major components: (1) sampling, (2) transcription, (3) analysis, and (4) interpretation. Our work on SALT provided solutions for the past problems with transcription format consistency and flexibility as well as standardization of many analyses. The major missing piece at this point was LSA data to help us interpret what constituted normal performance for children of a variety of ages under different speaking conditions.

DEVELOPING A REFERENCE DATABASE

To address the interpretation problem, we began to collect language samples from typically developing children in a collaborative effort with the MMSD in 1983. Subjects were randomly selected from schools located throughout the Madison district to ensure that they represented the range of socioeconomic status evident in Madison. To ensure that the broad range of "normal" performance was sampled, teachers were asked to judge those children in their classrooms who had no known disabilities as having high, average, or low oral communication skills. Ten children at each of these levels were subsequently selected for inclusion at each age level of the database. The current database thus includes language samples from 27 to 30 children at each of the ages of 3, 4, 5, 6, 7, 9, 11, and 13 years (Miller, 1990).

Language samples were collected from each of these children in two speaking contexts: (1) conversation and (2) narration. In the conversational context, the examiner asked the child a sequence of questions about family, activities, and so forth. In the narrative context, the child was asked to tell a favorite story, or to recount an episode from a favorite television program or movie. Narrative samples were obtained from the youngest children by asking them to tell a story about a picture from a fairy tale.

The decision to select these two speaking contexts was motivated by their educational relevance, usual clinical practice, and the amount of developmental data available for each. The conversational condition was selected because the majority of developmental data is based on conversations, either with parents or with examiners. In addition, conversational competence with adults was judged to be essential for educational progress, and this context was also consistent with the usual clinical practice of collecting language samples in adult–child conversations. Inclusion of the narrative speaking condition was motivated by the need to document children's progress in narration, a context relevant to acquiring reading skills and to relaying information in classrooms on a variety of topics. Narrative skills appear to develop throughout the childhood years, making them particularly useful in noting developmental progress. We also suspected that a narrative speaking context would place more pressure on the child, in terms of formulating spontaneous utterances, than would a conversational context.

Conversational and narrative language samples were audiorecorded from each of the 192 children participating in the Reference Database (RDB) project (Miller, 1990). These 384 language samples were transcribed into computer files by trained speech-language pathologists or research assistants using SALT transcription conventions. Standard analyses were run on each of these transcript files, with the results sent to a database for storage and summary statistical analysis.

Two versions of each transcript were analyzed. One version consisted of 100 complete and intelligible utterances; the second consisted of all utterances occurring in a 12-minute interval. By analyzing these two versions separately, we were able to quantify variables when the number of opportunities for production had been equated (in the 100-utterance version), as well as to document rate variables when the transcript durations had been equated (the 12-minute version). A summary of a number of RDB variables from the narrations produced by 9-year-old children appears in Table 1. This table lists the variable, the mean, the ±1 standard deviation (SD) range, the percentage of SD (% SD), and the range of raw scores. The percentage of SD (the SD for a variable divided by the mean) provides an index of the variability of a particular measure; the higher this number, the less stable the measure is for the age group.

The RDB represents the first large-scale attempt to conduct LSA on samples obtained under standard speaking contexts through this developmental period. The analysis of the RDB has led us to seek to distinguish between variables that mark developmental progress in language performance and variables that indicate disordered performance.

INDICES OF DEVELOPMENTAL PROGRESS

The RDB has revealed three indicators of developmental progress in the age range from 3 through 13 years. Each indexes a different aspect of language performance. The first, mean length of utterance (MLU) in morphemes, is a general index of syntactic progress that had previously been viewed as correlated with age only through approximately age 5 (Miller & Chapman, 1981). In addition to providing evidence that MLU is a useful developmental mea-

Table 1. Selected SALT measures from the 9-year-old *Reference Database* narrative samples ($N = 27$)

	Mean	SD	± 1 SD	% SD	Range
Content summary:					
100-utterance samples					
MLU	8.80	1.61	7.2–10.41	18	6.49–13.6
Total words	800	145	655–945	18	578–1,232
Different words	205	28	177–233	14	152–264
Utterances w/mazes	33	10	23–43	31	19–55
Bound morphemes					
Regular past	16	8	8–24	50	4–37
Plural	17	6	11–23	36	5–27
Possessive	6	4	2–10	73	1–14
Utterance content					
Personal pronouns					
Total	99	19	80–117	19	63–149
Types	9	1	8–10	13	7–11
Conjunctions					
Total	108	28	79–136	26	60–184
Types	7	1	5–8	20	4–9
Rate summary:					
12-minute samples					
Total utterances	184	34	150–219	19	110–282
Complete and intelligible	171	32	139–204	19	106–269
Total words	1,312	228	1,084–1,540	17	933–1,832
Different words	291	34	257–325	12	210–380

sure beyond age 5, the RDB has enabled us to add two new variables to our list of developmental indicators. One of these, the number of different words (DW) produced in 100 complete and intelligible utterances, represents an index of semantic diversity. The other, total number of words (TW) produced in a 12-minute sample, provides a general index of verbal productivity, encompassing such factors as speech motor maturation, utterance formulation skill, and word-finding skill. All of these measures have been found to be highly correlated with chronological age in children from 3 through 13 years of age (Miller, 1991b), suggesting that they can serve as useful measures of developmental progress in this age range.

INDICES OF DISORDERED PERFORMANCE

Analysis of the RDB has also suggested that "mazes" (defined by Loban, 1976, as false starts, repetitions, and reformulations) represent a possible index of language formulation or word-finding difficulty in children. We initially segregated mazes in our transcripts both to exclude them from MLU calculations and to measure their frequency in normally developing children. If children become more fluent as they get older, then mazes should decrease in frequency with increasing age. The RDB, however, suggests that these behaviors occur at a fairly high rate in speakers across this age range: 15% to 25%

of the utterances in the conversational samples contain mazes. In addition, mazes occurred in a higher proportion of utterances produced in the narration samples than in the conversational samples. Because of the increased utterance formulation load in the narrative context, these data suggest that mazes reflect formulation load. Further support for the use of mazes to index formulation load comes from the finding that mazes occurred more frequently in longer than in shorter utterances. We conclude that mazes will be a useful variable in attempting to document language formulation deficits in children.

Data from the RDB cannot be considered norms. We believe that language sample data cannot be normed in the psychometric sense, due to the large number of factors affecting children's performance that cannot be controlled (e.g., the examiner's interactive style). Clinical judgment still plays a large part in the interpretation of LSA data, beginning with determining whether the language sample reflects the child's usual performance. The RDB aids clinical judgment by providing information on the expected performance for a wide variety of measures in conversational and narrative speaking contexts.

LSA WITH DIVERSE POPULATIONS

The data reported above were collected only in Madison, Wisconsin, from an urban population less racially diverse (94% white in the 1980 census) than in many areas of the United States. The utility of the Madison RDB in interpreting the language produced by children from other geographic locations, or from other cultural groups, was unknown. To begin to address these questions, speech-language pathologists from the Cooperative Education Service Agency Number 9 (CESA-9) and members of the Language Analysis Laboratory in Madison have initiated a series of collaborative projects. The CESA-9, 1 of 12 intermediate education agencies in the state, is located in north central Wisconsin, where the school districts are primarily rural.

One project has focused on comparing rural and urban children on the three measures of developmental progress described above: (1) MLU, (2) number of DW in 100 complete and intelligible utterances, and (3) TW produced in 12-minute samples. CESA-9 speech-language pathologists collected conversational and narrative samples following the SALT protocol from 90 rural children, 30 each at the ages of 3, 5, and 7 years. SALT analyses of these samples revealed no statistically significant differences between these children and the Madison RDB children at these ages. Apparently, urban and rural children exhibit similar performance on these three productive language measures when age and sampling conditions are controlled. These findings have paved the way for a statewide LSA system (Miller, Freiberg, Rolland, & Reeves, 1990).

A second project has explored the use of the SALT protocol with Native American children from CESA-9. Conversational and narrative samples were collected from 14 Native American kindergarten children who spoke on one occasion to a Native American examiner, and on another occasion to a white examiner. Analyses of MLU, TW, and DW in the standard SALT speaking conditions revealed no differences according to speaking partner. However, these samples are currently being analyzed in more detail, in response to comments from the examiners involved in the project suggesting that there may be other culturally related differences in productive language performance. Further exploration of the impact of cultural differences on LSA data is clearly warranted; sampling conditions, topics, and interaction methods may need to be adjusted in order to draw valid conclusions about LSA results from nonwhite children.

USING SALT IN THE PUBLIC SCHOOL: A CASE STUDY

Some children perform well on standardized tests of language production but communicate poorly. Standardized tests may not reveal language production deficits such as utterance formulation problems or semantic referencing problems, especially when a child's comprehension skills are normal. SALT provides methods for documenting a variety of language production deficits that may not be captured through standardized tests or global language measures. We have chosen to illustrate these points by presenting a case study of a child whose oral language problems were not reflected in standardized tests and measures. SALT enabled us to analyze and interpret the data from this child in a new way.

HISTORICAL INFORMATION

Greg was an 8-year-old third grader on the caseload of one of the authors (MBR). He had begun receiving intensive treatment for expressive language and articula-

tion problems at age 2:6 (years:months). Intervention continued through kindergarten and first grade, when difficulties in reading began to emerge. He was evaluated by a multidisciplinary learning disabilities team, but no other academic or social problems were noted. He was reportedly well liked by his peers.

Greg had made significant gains in speech and language skills, progressing from almost completely unintelligible one-word utterances at age 3 to syntactically appropriate utterances with only minor residual articulation errors on /r/ and /l/ at age 6. However, language difficulties were still evident in third grade, and Greg was only reading at a preprimer level. Both parents and teachers observed that he tended to "ramble," and that his communication attempts were often difficult to follow. A battery of tests was administered in an effort to specify the nature of his language deficits.

Standardized tests suggested that Greg's cognitive and oral language comprehension skills were largely intact. He scored in the superior range on the Wechsler Intelligence Scale for Children-Revised (Wechsler, 1974), with a Verbal scale score of 125, a Performance scale score of 135, and a Full scale score of 134. His Peabody Picture Vocabulary Test-Revised (Dunn & Dunn, 1981) score placed him at the 60th percentile, but he scored at the 25th percentile on the Boehm Test of Basic Concepts (Boehm, 1971), during which he frequently asked "What do you mean?" Two of three comprehension subtests of the Test of Language Development-2 (TOLD-2) (Newcomer & Hammill, 1977) were within normal limits for his age, but his score of 8 on the Picture Vocabulary

subtest placed him below age expectations.

Greg's performance on standardized language production measures was more variable. He scored within normal limits on
two of three TOLD-2 production subtests,
but his score of 5 on the Sentence Imitation subtest revealed extreme difficulty in
repeating sentences. His performance on
the Test of Word Finding (German, 1986)
placed him at the 7th percentile, and
suggested "fast and inaccurate" naming
skills.

A SALT analysis revealed a type-token
ratio of .41 and an MLU of 7.25, placing
Greg within the range of performance of
the 9-year-olds in the RDB. However,
these general measures failed to reveal the
extent of his oral communication deficit.
More detailed SALT analyses were necessary in order to provide evidence that he
had an exceptional educational need requiring speech and language services.

SALT TRANSCRIPT

A portion of Greg's conversational sample can be found in Table 2. Reading the
transcript gives a sense of this child's
overall communication skills that is not
revealed by general measures such as
standardized tests or MLU. Even this
brief excerpt contains numerous examples
of mazes (e.g., lines 160, 173–174, 176–
177); word-finding difficulties (e.g., lines
162, 177, 179); and errors at various levels
(e.g., lines 165, 168, 171) that affect what
he is saying and how it sounds. The more
detailed SALT analysis described below
makes it possible to document these and
other phenomena that distinguish Greg's
language sample from RDB samples.

Table 2. A portion of Greg's conversational sample transcript

159	E	So what kinds of things do you get to eat at Ginza?
160	C	Well I only (I) went there once (and the)
161		and I ate chicken.
162	C	(Um what) What/'re those like Uncle Ben thing/s?
163	E	Rice?
164	C	Yeah rice and we put some stuff on it
165		what[EW:that] taste good [EU].
166	C	And the chicken too.
167	C	We put everything on it and I don't know
168		what a[EW:the] other stuff is called.
169	E	It was good though, huh?
170	C	Yes.
171	C	And they give[EW:gave] us the[EW:a] show.
172	C	They/'ll go like {boo boo boo boo} for a little.
173	C	(They/'ll ju*) Juggle/ing (um) the pepper
174		shaker (and the salt sha*) and (sh*) salt.
175	E	Do they do anything else?
176	C	(N*) No, (they throw) if you have (um)
177		shrimp they/'ll throw the (um) crab thing/s.
178	C	You know what.
179	C	The pincher thing/s.
180	C	They/'ll throw it[EW:them] at (me) peo-ple.
181	C	And they throw (um) >
182	C	(At our) when I went they throw[EW:threw] (um)
183	C	What you call it [EU].

Note. E = examiner utterance; C = child utterance; EW = word
error; EU = utterance error. Mazes appear in parentheses; slashes
indicate bound morpheme contexts. Asterisks indicate absent or
incomplete units.

SALT ANALYSIS SUMMARY

Table 3 shows Greg's LSA data on an
abbreviated SALT summary form developed by the MMSD speech-language pathologists to provide a clinically useful
summary of a child's SALT analysis along
with the relevant RDB data to aid interpretation. Greg's age placed him between the

Table 3. SALT analysis summary: Greg's conversation as compared with 9-year-olds ($N = 27$) in the Madison reference database

Measure	Student	Mean	SD	+/− 1 SD	Range
I. Timing					
# Utterances/min	13.10	15.11	2.54	12.57–17.86	8.67–20.75
# Words/min	82.38	88.41	22.27	66.14–110.68	36.0–137.42
II. Intelligibility					
% Complete & intelligible	91.82	92.35	4.53	87.83–96.88	80.65–99.01
III. Mazes & overlaps					
# Utterances w/mazes	34	25	8	17–33	9–42
IV. Semantics					
Total words	651	592	94	498–686	431–742
Different words	208	209	26	183–235	167–278
V. Word lists*	Greg's data all within normal limits.				
VI. Syntax/morphology					
MLU-morphemes	7.25	6.50	1.04	5.46–7.54	4.62–8.32
VII. Bound morphemes[†]	Greg's data all within normal limits.				
VIII. Errors	Greg made 13 word-level and 21 utterance-level errors.				

*Includes questions, negatives, conjunctions, modals, and personal pronouns.
[†]Includes plural; present progressive; regular past; possessive; third-person singular present tense.

RDB data for 7-year-olds and 9-year-olds; the decision to use the RDB 9-year-olds as a reference group was made on the basis of his overall developmental level, as described below. The data from Greg's conversational sample appear in the "Student" column. The RDB data are in the same form as in Table 1 with the analyses organized into eight categories. A number of more detailed analyses in each section have been omitted from this summary form.

On the timing and speech intelligibility measures in Sections I and II, Greg's performance placed him within normal limits according to the RDB data. However, as shown in Section III, 34 of Greg's utterances contained mazes, placing him slightly more than 1 SD above the mean. Further analysis of the 52 mazes he produced revealed that only 9 consisted of the simple interjection "um." Instead, 16 of Greg's mazes were repetitions, and 27 were revisions. Twenty of these revisions were at the phrase level. Such revisions suggest that Greg has difficulty organizing his conversational utterances, either because of word-finding problems or problems in formulating larger utterance constituents. These revisions undoubtedly make Greg difficult to follow.

Greg's performance on the semantic, morphological, and syntactic measures in Sections IV, V, VI, and VII was within normal limits. It is interesting to note that Greg's MLU approaches 1 SD above the mean for 9-year-olds. In our clinical experience, relatively large MLUs often characterize children exhibiting word-finding or utterance formulation problems.

As summarized in Section VIII of the form, Greg produced 34 errors in his sample, with 13 of these at the word level and the remaining 21 at the utterance level. In our clinical experience with the RDB samples, such errors are extremely rare, especially in children more than 5 years of age. Further, most of Greg's utterance-level errors resulted in utterances that were incomplete or ambiguous, making them extremely difficult for the listener to interpret.

In summary, Greg presented a profile of performance in which he performed within normal limits on standardized measures of language performance and the general developmental variables from LSA (e.g., MLU). However, the detailed SALT analysis of error categories revealed significant production deficits. He has significant difficulty producing clear and coherent messages despite his apparently adequate knowledge of the language system. His problems appear to be with accessing his knowledge to formulate messages. Clinical judgment supported by the frequency of his word-level errors; his frequent failures to specify subject, verb, or object in utterance-level errors; and the maze analysis results suggest that word finding is the cause of his production deficit.

IMPLEMENTING LSA IN THE SCHOOLS

The MMSD has been through various stages of implementation of the SALT program in its schools. The first stage of implementation that was both cost-effective and functional was identifying and training a core group of interested speech-language pathologists to function as mentors, or a support group, for the rest of the district. These individuals received train-

ing in the transcription, analysis, and interpretation procedures of the program and then began to teach the procedures to other district speech-language pathologists. This strategy provided the district with a set of "peer experts" able to field questions from speech-language pathologists and to distribute training to small regional groups.

After the training of a core SALT group, the various options for the most cost-effective way to implement the program in a district must be reviewed. Decisions about who will have the responsibility for transcribing the tape-recorded language samples, and who will conduct the analyses of the samples, are among those to be made. Because of the amount of SLP time required to transcribe a tape (1.5–2 hours), we have experimented with having the samples transcribed by trained typists or university students. Although this strategy allows a greater proportion of the SLP's time to be spent on interpreting the data and performing more detailed analyses, it also has several disadvantages. Nonprofessional transcribers must be trained to segment, transcribe, and code utterances reliably. In addition, if the interval between the time when the tape is submitted for transcribing and the time when it is received back is too lengthy, the SLP may forget some of the interaction, making it impossible to add this information to the transcript or report. Finally, even with this option, the SLP must still review the transcript to correct errors and to ensure that the tape is an accurate reflection of the recording.

The cost of having speech-language pathologists transcribe their own tapes must be weighed against several advantages of this option, which are not easily measured in dollars and cents. In transcribing their own samples, speech-language pathologists can add commentary regarding nonverbal responses and comments by the students, and samples may be more intelligible to them because they were there during the interaction. Similarly, the more detailed picture of a student that the speech-language pathologist develops through being involved in transcription cannot be overlooked. While transcribing the sample, the speech-language pathologist cannot help but begin to form hypotheses about the student's language performance. Analysis and interpretation begin long before the "print" of the transcript is ready. Through transcription, the speech-language pathologist is also likely to become more aware of the interactions in the data, for example, the relationship of pauses and mazes to word retrieval and formulation difficulties, to MLU, to the use of nonspecific words, and so forth.

The ideal situation, which we have not yet achieved, may be a combination of these two strategies. In this scenario, a typist would be trained to provide a first-level transcription of the sample. A computer disk containing the transcript file would be returned to the speech-language pathologist, who would listen to and correct the sample while reading it on his or her own computer screen. The speech-language pathologist would then analyze and print the transcript file and the relevant analysis tables. Although this strategy requires that each speech-language pathologist have a computer, we would argue that the advantages of having speech-language pathologists spend relatively more of their time in analysis, interpreta-

tion, and development of focused intervention programs will prove cost-effective in the long run.

LSA AND A CHANGING VIEW OF LANGUAGE DISORDER

Implementing LSA in school settings has, more than anything else, caused us to reconsider our conceptualization of language impairment. Language-impaired children have been categorized in several different ways, primarily involving differences in their comprehension and production skills. The DSM-III-R (American Psychiatric Association, 1987) identifies two groups: (1) those with comprehension and production deficits and (2) those with production-only deficits. Tallal (1988) distinguished three groups: (1) those with comprehension delayed relative to production, (2) those with both comprehension and production delays, and (3) those with delays only in production. Rapin (1988) defined three different categories: (1) expressive disorders with normal comprehension, (2) mixed disorders with impaired articulation, and (3) higher-order processing disorders. These categorizations focus on the independence of comprehension and production and are primarily defined by developmental variables. Recent work suggests that these categories may be too broad. Rather than viewing comprehension and production as unitary constructs, the different levels of linguistic performance (i.e., phonology, vocabulary, syntax, semantics, and pragmatics) should be differentiated within each (Bates & Thal, 1991; Nelson, 1991; Snow, 1991).

In general, language-disordered children show a later onset of language skills and a slower rate of acquisition; some never achieve the language skills of their peers (Aram, Ekelman, & Nation, 1984; Schery, 1985; Weiner, 1985). There is an increasing recognition that language impairment is not a unitary construct, and multidimensional models of development and disorder must be used to document different disorder types (Fletcher, 1991; Miller, 1987, 1991a; Snow, 1991; Tallal, 1988). The research literature is beginning to catch up with what clinicians dealing with language-impaired children have known for some time: There are several types of impaired language performances that can be clinically defined. Although the boundaries between these types are not completely distinct, a better description of the types will aid our quest for improved service to these children. The clinical message is that children labeled "language disordered" exhibit very different language skills; treatments must be differentiated accordingly.

While participating in the LSA project, a group of master speech-language pathologists from the MMSD were asked to describe their perception of distinct types of impaired language performances. There was a great deal of uniformity in their responses, with six different types of language production impairment defined by the group. Table 4 summarizes the clinical typology of language impairment along with the LSA measurement categories associated with each type. There is one category for developmental delays and six different types of "disordered" performance generally defined by different error patterns.

Several of these disorder types correspond to descriptions beginning to emerge in the literature, including utterance formulation problems and word-finding defi-

Table 4. A clinical typology of language production disorders

Clinical types	LSA measurement categories
Disorders	
Utterance formulation	False starts, repetitions, and reformulations of phrase or clause-level units; pauses within and between utterances; word-order errors
Word finding	Pauses within utterances, false starts or reformulations of single words, word repetitions, word omissions, and substitutions
Rate: Hypoverbal	Decreased numbers of utterances and words per minute, pauses within and between utterances
Rate: Hyperverbal	Increased numbers of utterances and words per minute, possible combination with reduced semantic content
Pragmatic/discourse	Noncontingent utterances, poor topic maintenance, inadequate pronominal reference and introduction of new information, poor narrative structure
Semantic/reference	Overgeneralization and word choice errors; incomplete utterances, noun-phrase-verb phrase asymmetry; redundancy
Delay	Mean length of utterance; number of different words; total number of words; syntactic measures, e.g., NP, VP, negatives, questions, and complex sentence forms

Note. Adapted from Miller (1987, 1991b). Early versions of this table were based on an ongoing project with speech-language clinicians of the Madison Metropolitan School District.

cits. Two categories, semantic/reference problems and pragmatic/discourse problems, are very broad, and clinical consensus is that there is a variety of different patterns of performance for each of these types. Only improved measurement and description of disordered performance will improve the specificity of the semantic and pragmatic disorder categories. The rate category is also of interest. We have long recognized that many language-impaired children do not talk as much as their normal peers, but we have not used this information to aim interventions toward increasing rates of verbal output. Instead, low rates of utterance and word production have been viewed as hindrances to treatment programs focused on increasing syntactic complexity in production. Our group's clinical experience suggests that communicative effectiveness can sometimes be greatly improved by increasing the number of communicative attempts, even when these are less than perfect. Other rate problems include excessively long pauses between and within utterances, which may result in a child being viewed as "willful" or "uncooperative." Such children may be actually suffering from severe word-finding or utterance formulation problems; they may have adopted a strategy of pausing rather than talking their way through difficulties and producing frequent mazes. There are a few children who talk too rapidly, producing messages with very little content. These children tax the listener's comprehension skills to the point that no one wants to talk with them. It is almost as if the increased rate is used to compensate for the lack of message content, that is, as an adaptive strategy to help them hold the floor.

Because the measurement categories for these disorder types are not distinct, there is a clinical art to identifying and describing language impairment, as well as a science. The picture we have painted so far clearly indicates that the science is far from complete. We can be encouraged, however, by the increased recognition of the complexity of the problem and the development of assessment tools, such as LSA, that will allow us to describe developmental progress as well as deficits in performance.

Although the focus of this article has been on language production, we do not intend to minimize the importance of language comprehension to language and communication development—quite the contrary. We begin with production because it is accessible; solving the behavioral categorization and measurement problems in production may aid the more difficult problem of quantifying the largely private event of language comprehension.

•   •   •

Our experience suggests that LSA is crucial to identifying and describing disordered language performance. A number of important diagnostic features of language production, such as vocabulary diversity, can only be determined feasibly through computer LSA techniques. Finally, LSA suggests categories of disordered performance that expand the current conceptualization of language impairment as delayed acquisition in important ways. We are fast approaching the age when it will be imperative for school clinicians to have portable computers enabling access to computerized LSA for identifying, describing, and monitoring intervention services to children with productive language deficits.

REFERENCES

American Psychiatric Association. (1987). *Diagnostic and statistical manual of mental disorders* (3rd ed., rev.). Washington, DC: Author.

Aram, D., Ekelman, B., & Nation, J. (1984). Preschoolers with language disorders: Ten years later. *Journal of Speech and Hearing Research, 27*, 232–244.

Bates, E., & Thal, D. (1991). Associations and dissociations in child language development. In J. Miller (Ed.), *Research in child language disorders: A decade of progress*. Boston, MA: College Hill Press.

Boehm, A. (1971). *Boehm test of basic concepts*. New York, NY: The Psychological Corporation.

Dunn, L., & Dunn, L. (1981). *Peabody Picture Vocabulary Test* (rev.). Circle Pines, MN: American Guidance Service.

Fletcher, P. (1991). Evidence from syntax for language impairment. In J. Miller (Ed.), *Research on child language disorders: A decade of progress*. Boston, MA: College Hill Press.

German, D. (1986). *Test of word finding*. Allen Park, TX: DLM.

Loban, W. (1976). *Language development: kindergarten through grade twelve* (Research Rep. No. 18). National Council of Teachers of English. Urbana, IL.

Miller, J. (1987). A grammatical characterization of language disorder. *Proceedings of the First International Symposium on Specific Speech and Language Disorders in Children*. London, England: AFASIC Press.

Miller, J. (1990). *The SALT reference database*. Madison, WI: University of Wisconsin-Madison, Waisman Center, Language Analysis Laboratory.

Miller, J. (1991a). Research on child language disorders: A progress report. In J. Miller (Ed.), *Research on child language disorders: A decade of progress*. Boston, MA: College Hill Press.

Miller, J. (1991b). Quantifying productive language disorder. In J. Miller (Ed.), *Research on child language disorders: A decade of progress*. Boston, MA: College Hill Press.

Miller, J., & Chapman, R. (1981). The relation between age and mean length of utterance in morphemes. *Journal of Speech and Hearing Research, 24*, 154–161.

Miller, J., & Chapman, R. (1982). *SALT: Systematic analysis of language transcripts-Harris computer version* [Computer program]. Madison, WI: University of Wisconsin-Madison, Waisman Center, Language Analysis Laboratory.

Miller, J., Freiberg, C., Rolland, M., & Reeves, M. (1990, November). *Implementing computerized language samples analysis in the public school*. Paper presented at the annual convention of the American Speech-Language-Hearing Association, Seattle, WA.

Nelson, K. (1991). Event knowledge and the development of language function. In J. Miller (Ed.), *Research on child language disorders: A decade of progress*. Boston, MA: College Hill Press.

Newcomer, P., & Hammill, D. (1977). *Test of language development-2*. Austin, TX: Pro-Ed.

Rapin, I. (1988). Discussion. In J. Kavanagh & T. Truss (Eds.), *Learning disabilities: Proceedings of the national conference*. Parkton, MD: York Press.

Schery, T. (1985). Correlates of language development in language-disordered children. *Journal of Speech and Hearing Disorders, 50*, 73–83.

Snow, C. (1991). Diverse conversational contexts for the acquisition of various language skills. In J. Miller (Ed.), *Research on child language disorders: A decade of progress*. Boston, MA: College Hill Press.

Tallal, P. (1988). Developmental language disorders. In J. Kavanagh & T. Truss (Eds.), *Learning disabilities: Proceedings of the National Conference*. Parkton, MD: York Press.

Wechsler, D. (1974). *Wechsler Intelligence Scale for Children* (rev.). New York, NY: The Psychological Corporation.

Weiner, P. (1985). The value of follow-up studies. *Topics in Language Disorders, 5*, 78–92.

Part III
Language Assessment of Some of the More Severely Language Impaired

Literacy and augmentative and alternative communication (AAC): The expectations and priorities of parents and teachers

Janice Light, PhD
Assistant Professor
Department of Communication Disorders
The Pennsylvania State University

David McNaughton, MSc
Doctoral Student
Department of Educational and School
    Psychology and Special Education
The Pennsylvania State University
University Park, Pennsylvania

IT IS WELL recognized that students who use augmentative and alternative communication (AAC) systems are "at risk" for the development of functional literacy skills (Kelford Smith, Thurston, Light, Parnes, & O'Keefe, 1989; Koppenhaver & Yoder, 1990; McNaughton & Tawney, in press). Without functional literacy skills, individuals who use AAC systems are severely restricted in their access to educational and vocational opportunities. The challenge in the next decade is to identify strategies to overcome these difficulties so that functional literacy outcomes become a reality for a greater number of students who use AAC systems. To do this, a clear understanding of the factors that contribute to successful literacy must be developed.

The research with nondisabled populations identifying significant determinants of literacy acquisition has examined many different factors (e.g., instructional variables, student characteristics). Recent findings have highlighted the importance of

Top Lang Disord, 1993,13(2),33–46
© 1993 Aspen Publishers, Inc.

high expectations of parents and teachers as one factor that influences a student's progress in reading and writing development (Cooper, 1979; Durkin, 1984; Palardy, 1969; Parsons, Adler, & Kaczala, 1982). As Good and Brophy (1984) noted, "our expectations affect the way we behave, and the way we behave affects how other people respond" (p. 98). Most of what we know about parents' and teachers' expectations and literacy development is drawn from research with speaking, nondisabled students who were at risk for literacy development (e.g., low socioeconomic status, single-parent home). To date, there have only been a few studies that have directly addressed expectations for literacy development for students using AAC. The intent of this article is to provide a brief overview of the research on literacy expectations for students without disabilities, to report the results of the research to date on expectations and priorities for students using AAC systems, to discuss implications of the research results for education and clinical practice, and to suggest directions for future research.

EXPECTATIONS FOR LITERACY DEVELOPMENT IN NONDISABLED INDIVIDUALS

The importance of both parent and teacher expectations for a student's literacy achievement has been well documented in research with nondisabled individuals (for reviews, see Good & Brophy, 1984; Seginer, 1983). Expectations have typically been measured through parent and teacher report of expected academic performance, years of school, report card grades, and future occupation. Thompson, Alexander, and Entwhistle (1988) examined the effect of parental expectations on reading achievement (as measured by standardized tests) for first-grade students. Although the children of parents with high and low expectations began school with similar early reading scores, the children of parents with high expectations demonstrated significantly greater progress throughout the year. Teacher expectations also have an impact on a student's progress in literacy instruction. In an early study, Palardy (1969) identified two groups of first-grade teachers. The first group of teachers ($n = 10$) thought that boys could learn to read as successfully as girls; the second group ($n = 14$) thought girls would demonstrate more benefit from instruction. There were no initial differences in the achievement levels of boys and girls at the start of the school year. Testing in March, however, revealed that in classes where teachers did not think boys could learn as well as girls, the boys had lower standardized reading achievement scores. In classes in which the teachers held equal expectations for boys and girls, the boys slightly outscored the girls. The expectation of some teachers that boys would make less progress appeared to result in a self-fulfilling prophecy of diminished accomplishment.

Nevertheless, it is not entirely clear how parent and teacher expectations are formed. Seginer (1983) suggested three antecedents to parental expectations: (1) school feedback, (2) parental aspirations, and (3) parental knowledge of their child's development and performance. The research suggests that parent and teacher expectations influence student performance in two main ways. First, expectations directly influence the priority given to literacy activities, and hence influence the quantity and quality of opportunities for participation in literacy activities provided for students both at home and at school. Second, the expectations of parents and teachers can be communicated directly or indirectly to the student, and thereby affect the student's own expectancy of success, in turn influencing the student's motivation in learning. The belief that an academic goal is achievable (and worth achieving) can influence the effort and perseverance that a student demonstrates in an educational program (Cohen, McDonell, & Osborn, 1989; Parsons & Ruble, 1977).

OPPORTUNITIES FOR PARTICIPATION

Parents with high expectations for literacy development often consider reading and writing a priority and act on this belief by providing their children with access to reading materials and adult assistance with reading activities at home (Durkin, 1984; Goldenberg, 1984; Thompson et al., 1988). In contrast, low expectations or a low parental priority for literacy acquisition may result in limited reading opportunities in the home. In examining the factors that lead to progress in literacy acquisition for children traditionally considered to be at risk for literacy development, both Durkin (1984) and Goldenberg (1984) emphasized the importance of an interested, supportive adult in the home.

At school, it has been found that students perceived as low achievers are offered substantially different opportunities to participate than are students for whom

teachers hold high expectations of success (Brattesani, Weinstein, & Marshall, 1984; Cooper, 1979). Students viewed as low achievers typically are provided with fewer opportunities to respond; furthermore, when they are asked to participate, they are given less time to respond (Good & Brophy, 1984). These instructional techniques may lead to less student success, not more. As noted earlier, the expectations for low achievement may become a self-fulfilling prophecy (Palardy, 1969). In contrast, teacher behaviors associated with high expectations (e.g., more opportunities to participate, longer wait time for responses) have been found to increase both the accuracy and frequency of responses by individuals with disabilities (Harris, 1982; Lee, 1985).

STUDENT EXPECTATIONS OF SUCCESS

Students who believe they can be successful at a task are more likely to persevere and produce higher quality work than students who do not have the same expectations for a positive outcome (Cohen et al., 1989; Parsons & Ruble, 1977). Parental and teacher expectations can be powerful influences in determining students' perceptions of their own capabilities and their expectations for success. In an investigation of factors affecting student expectations of success, Parsons and colleagues (1982) reported that parental expectations can have a greater impact on the students' views of their own abilities than the students' actual records of educational achievement.

With respect to the role of expectations in the classroom, research by Brattesani and colleagues (1984) has demonstrated that students are aware that teachers behave differently when they have low expectations for student achievement than they do when they have high expectations for success. Students' perceptions of teachers' behaviors and intentions may motivate and direct student behaviors (Brattesani et al., 1984; Braun, 1976; Cooper, 1979). When teachers expect limited progress, students may themselves adopt diminished expectations for success, affecting both their motivation and effort.

The expectations held by parents, educators, and students form a tangled web of potential influences on literacy outcomes (Brattesani et al., 1984; Braun, 1976; Parsons et al., 1982). These expectations can play a critical role in determining an individual's reading and writing progress: negative expectations can impede progress; positive expectations can serve to facilitate development. Clearly, high expectations alone are not enough to guarantee the successful acquisition of literacy skills; both informal and formal literacy activities also play a critical role (Dunn, 1981; Goldenberg, 1984; Seginer, 1983). In the absence of positive expectations, however, both the quantity and quality of these experiences will be severely affected.

EXPECTATIONS FOR LITERACY DEVELOPMENT IN STUDENTS WHO USE AAC SYSTEMS

A number of persons who use AAC systems and have achieved high levels of literacy have reported retrospectively that they attribute their success in learning to read and write, at least in part, to the positive expectations and support of family members and others (e.g., Brown, 1954; Koppenhaver, Evans, & Yoder, 1991; McNaughton, 1991). These reports suggest that positive expectations and support from others may be one factor that contributes to successful literacy outcomes for students using AAC.

Light, Koppenhaver, Lee, and Riffle (1992), in conjunction with the Augmentative Communication Service at the Hugh MacMillan Rehabilitation Centre in Ontario, Canada, and the Pennsylvania Assistive Technology Center in the United States, conducted a survey of parents and teachers to explore the home and school literacy experiences of students who use AAC systems. Sixty-nine students were represented in the study, ranging in age from 3 to 21 years, with a mean age of 13 years. The majority of the students had cerebral palsy (71%); other disabilities reported included mental retardation, visual impairment, hearing impairment, and traumatic brain injury. Students with severe and profound cognitive impairments were not included in the study. The students used multiple means to communicate: 68% used gestures and signs, 51% used a voice output communication system, 50% used nonelectronic communication displays, and 41% used some speech or speech approximations.

Parental expectations

A total of 66 parents responded to the survey. These parents were asked to report on the students' current skills in reading and writing. According to parent report, current skill levels varied across the sample. The majority of students were not functionally literate at the time of the survey. Only 9 of the 59 students over the age of 9 (15%) were reported to be able to read the newspaper or more complex texts.

Parents were also asked to indicate the level of literacy skills they expected their children to attain by age 25. The level of skills expected at age 25 by parents varied across the sample. Approximately 48% of the parents expected their children to achieve functional literacy skills (i.e., the ability to read the newspaper or more complex texts). In contrast, approximately 8% of the parents expected that their children would not learn to read and write and 31% expected that they would learn to read and write only a limited number of words.

Most parents (62%) anticipated that their children's literacy skills would improve by age 25; however, a significant number of parents (24%) indicated that they did not expect any improvement in their children's current skill levels by age 25. Thus, it seems that although most parents had positive expectations for progress in literacy learning, there was still a significant number of parents who did not expect any improvement in reading and writing skills. Given the design of the study, it was not possible to determine if parental expectations were "realistic" or not. However, it is important to note that low expectations for development in literacy achievement may result in reduced emphasis on literacy-related experiences in the home environment. The reduced opportunity to be involved in literacy-related activities may, in turn, have a negative impact on literacy achievement, resulting in a self-fulfilling prophecy.

Also of interest in the survey was the fact that nine parents (14%) indicated that they had no idea what to expect in terms of literacy development for their children by age 25. Typically, parents of children with disabilities have had minimal (if any) exposure to people with disabilities prior to the birth of their own child or the onset of their child's disability (Featherstone, 1980). As a result, they have minimal experience on which to base their expectations for their children's future development. This problem may be especially acute with a low-incidence population such as the AAC population. Many parents may lack the information necessary to develop realistic expectations for their children's future development.

Teacher expectations

Light and colleagues (1992) also surveyed the teachers of the students to investigate teacher expectations for literacy development. Forty-one teachers responded to the survey. These teachers were asked the same questions as parents: to report on the students' current level of literacy skills, and to indicate their expectations for the students' literacy performance at age 25. The students' current skill levels, as reported by teachers, varied across the sample. Teachers' judgments of their students' skills were congruent with parents' judgments for 51% of the students. For 35% of the students, teachers reported higher levels of achievement than did parents, whereas for 14%, they reported lower skill levels.

As with the parents, the literacy outcomes expected at age 25 varied across the sample. The majority of teachers (64%) expected that their students would achieve functional literacy skills by age 25. Teacher expectations for future achievement were congruent with parent expectations in only

33% of the cases. Teacher expectations were lower than parent expectations in 47% of the cases. Most of the teachers (73%) expected their students' reading and writing skills to improve by age 25; 24% expected no improvement. Given the nature of the study, it is not possible to ascertain whether the expectations held by parents and/or teachers were realistic. Further longitudinal research is required to determine the impact of expectations and other factors (e.g., type and intensity of instruction) on literacy outcomes.

PRIORITIES FOR STUDENTS WHO USE AAC SYSTEMS

Obviously, positive expectations are not sufficient to ensure the successful attainment of literacy skills. Functional reading and writing skills are not automatically acquired without instruction (Herriman, 1986). Positive expectations can, however, create the impetus for effective instruction (Goldenberg, 1984; Seginer, 1983). It is therefore important to understand not only the expectations of parents and teachers, but also the priority accorded to literacy learning by parents and teachers. The importance attached to literacy learning will influence the time and effort given to formal instruction and to informal literacy-related activities. Two studies (Light & Kelford Smith, in press; Light et al., 1992) provide some insight into the value accorded to literacy learning for students who use AAC systems.

Parental priorities

Light and Kelford Smith (in press) conducted a survey to compare the home literacy experiences of physically disabled preschoolers who use AAC systems to the experiences of their nondisabled peers. Questionnaires were completed by 15 parents in each group. The children ranged in age from 2 to 6 years. Children in the AAC group all had a primary diagnosis of a physical disability, and all required AAC systems. Children in the nondisabled group had no known physical, sensory, and/or speech and language impairments. Parents in the two groups were asked to rank order, on a scale of 1 to 8, various activities (feeding, toilet training, dressing, independent mobility, communicating, learning to read, learning to write, and making friends), indicating the importance of the activity for their children at the time of the study.

Learning to communicate effectively was considered to be the most important priority by the parents in the AAC group (median rank = 1). Next priority was given to independent mobility (median rank = 4), feeding (median rank = 4.5), toilet training (median rank = 5), and making friends (median rank = 5.5). Lowest priority was given to learning to read (median rank = 6) and learning to write (median rank = 6.5). Parents of the nondisabled children gave highest priority to making friends (median rank = 2) and communicating effectively (median rank = 2). Learning to read (median rank = 4), learning to write (median rank = 5), and dressing (median rank = 5) were considered to be next most important. Lowest priority was given to toilet training (median rank = 7), feeding skills (median rank = 7), and independent mobility (median rank = 8), perhaps because these goals had been attained successfully or because development in these areas seemed to be progressing satisfactorily.

Most interesting, in the context of this article, was the priority given to reading and writing by the two groups of parents. The parents of the nondisabled children considered reading and writing to be important priorities, second only to making friends and learning to communicate effectively. For the parents in the AAC group, however, these activities were considered to be the lowest priority. This is not to say that these parents felt that reading and writing were not important, but rather the results indicate that the parents believed that these skills were less important for their children than learning to communicate effectively and learning various self-help skills. The priorities expressed by parents of the AAC children seem to have been influenced by developmental priorities and by the desire to maximize their children's independence. When communication and self-help skills are successfully acquired, caregiving demands will be decreased, and the children will realize greater independence.

It is important to recognize, however, that since reading and writing are considered to be of lesser importance than other areas of skill development, parents may give less attention to literacy activities. The early literacy experiences of preschoolers who use AAC systems may be quantitatively and qualitatively different from those of their nondisabled peers (Light & Kelford Smith, in press). These different experiential bases may affect subsequent literacy learning in school.

Light and associates (1992) also addressed the issue of priorities for skill development in their study of the home and school literacy experiences of students between the ages of 3 and 21. In this study, parents and teachers were asked to indicate the top three priorities for their students who use AAC systems from the following list of activities: learning self-help skills (feeding, toileting, dressing, mobility); developing vocational skills; making friends; learning to read; learning to write; communicating effectively; developing world knowledge; and developing recreational interests and skills.

Communicating effectively was considered to be one of the top three priorities by 77% of the 66 parents who responded to the survey. Learning self-help skills was selected as a top priority by 47% of the parents. Learning to read was identified by 41% of the parents. Learning to write was considered to be less important than learning to read by most parents; fewer than 25% of the parents selected this activity as one of their three top priorities.

The top priorities identified by parents in the Light and colleagues (1992) study were very similar to those identified by the parents of preschoolers using AAC systems in the Light and Kelford Smith (in press) study, despite the fact that the mean age of the children in the former study was 13 years compared to a mean age of 4 years in the Light and Kelford Smith study.

Teacher priorities

Light and colleagues (1992) also asked the 41 teachers in their study to indicate the three activities that they felt were priorities for their students within their educational programs. Communicating effectively was considered to be a top priority by the majority of the teachers (93%). Learning to read (selected by 63% of the teachers) was the second most frequently selected priority, while learning to write was the third most frequently selected activity (selected by 44% of the teachers). Teachers were more apt to consider reading and writing to be priorities than were parents. Both teachers and parents tended to value learning to read more than learning to write.

The number one priority identified by teachers was congruent with the top priority indicated by parents in only 47% of the cases. Most parents and teachers did not agree on which goal was most important for the students using AAC.

EDUCATIONAL AND CLINICAL IMPLICATIONS

Historically, the multidisciplinary teams that provide services to students with severe communication disabilities have tended to focus on issues of face-to-face communication and issues of access to assistive technology. More recently, there has been a growing recognition that, in order to be optimally effective, these teams also need to address issues of literacy development (Blackstone, 1989; Koppenhaver & Yoder, 1990). Given what we know to date regarding expectations and priorities for literacy development, what directions are indicated in educational and clinical practice with students who use AAC? The research suggests the importance of the issues discussed in greater detail in the following sections.

Assessing the environment for literacy learning

Given the embryonic state of knowledge about literacy issues in the AAC field, there are no clear-cut guidelines for con-

ducting assessments of reading and writing skills and for planning intervention. To date, the focus of literacy assessment and intervention with learners who use AAC systems has been on the learners themselves and their current skills. However, given the potential role of parent, teacher, and learner expectations and priorities in influencing literacy outcomes, it seems reasonable to argue that assessment and intervention should extend beyond the consideration of learner skills in isolation and also consider the broader environment for literacy learning.

Parents, teachers, other professionals, and students themselves may be interviewed or asked to complete written questionnaires to determine their expectations for literacy development. Parents, professionals, and students may also be asked to report their priorities from a list of relevant goals and activities. Observations in the classroom and home may be used to confirm and supplement parent, teacher, and student report. These observations will provide valuable information about the quantity and quality of literacy-related activities and instruction.

Fostering positive and appropriate expectations

The study by Light and colleagues (1992) suggests that there are still a significant number of parents and teachers who have minimal expectations for their children to make any progress in learning to read or write. Low expectations for development may translate into a neglect of literacy-related activities and ultimately into a self-fulfilling prophecy of limited achievement. Therefore, the first step to intervention should be to foster positive attitudes toward literacy learning for students who use AAC systems, their parents, and their teachers.

Expectations for progress in reading and writing should be positive, but they should also be realistic. According to Good and Brophy (1984), "expectations should be appropriate rather than necessarily 'high,' and they must be followed by ... learning experiences that move the students through the curriculum at a pace they can handle" (p. 110). Care should be taken to ensure that both short- and long-term goals are identified so that parents, teachers, and students can expect and achieve high rates of success.

In many cases, parents, teachers, and students themselves may lack the information necessary to develop realistic expectations for the students' future literacy development. Concerted efforts must be made to disseminate available information about the emergence of literacy skills for students using AAC; continued research is required to further understanding of the development of reading and writing skills.

Students who use AAC systems, their parents, and support professionals may have had limited access to others who have similar disabilities and who have achieved successful literacy outcomes. They may have had only minimal exposure, if any, to models of successful literacy learners who use AAC. Yet the research with nondisabled students suggests that models can play an especially important role in the development of expectations (Picou & Carter, 1976).

Intervention to support literacy development may need to extend beyond direct instruction with the student using AAC systems and also provide education for parents and other facilitators. The goal of parent education should be to empower parents with the knowledge and skills that they require to support their children's literacy development. Parents require knowledge and skills in a number of areas: an understanding of their children's current skills, clear and realistic goals for both short-term and long-term development, and strategies to reach the identified goals.

Providing a map for literacy learning

Marriner, Yorkston, Dowden, and Dudgeon (1989) suggested the analogy of a road map to describe the types of information that facilitators require to support the communication development of persons using AAC systems. This same analogy can be applied to literacy learning. First, parents and other facilitators must know their current location. What are their children's current reading and writing skills? What are their children's strengths? What areas require remediation? Second, parents must have a final destination as a goal. They must be motivated to reach this destination and must feel that the final destination is achievable. Parents need to develop realistic expectations for their children's future literacy development and must have a clear understanding of why literacy development is important for their children. Third, parents need to be able to recognize landmarks en route to their final destination. These landmarks will allow parents to judge progress toward their destination or final goal and to determine if the journey is unfolding as expected.

Learning to read and write is a complex process and one that may require a significant amount of time for many learners. If parents have a clear sense of the milestones en route to the attainment of literacy skills, they will be better able to keep track of their children's progress. Finally, parents also need to be aware of potential hazards or indications that their course has strayed from the planned route so that they can look for assistance to reestablish their intended direction. There may be times when children do not seem to be making progress in learning to read and write. Intervention approaches may need to be reevaluated to ensure that instruction is effective. Parents need to be able to recognize when their children are encountering problems and seek help from professionals with the necessary expertise. With a well-drawn map delineating their children's current literacy skills, expectations for future development, and signposts and potential hazards, parents will be better equipped to support their children in achieving successful literacy outcomes.

Providing preservice and inservice training for teachers

In addition to educating parents of children who use AAC systems, it is also necessary to ensure that teachers and other professionals have access to the information and resources they require to support the literacy development of their students. Interest in literacy issues has grown in recent years; however, knowledge of literacy development for learners who use AAC systems is still limited. There is an urgent need for ongoing research to address literacy issues in order to extend the empirical knowledge base. There is also an urgent need for effective dissemination of the information that is currently available. Professionals should be encouraged to share research findings

and clinical and educational experiences in publications and presentations.

Most of the current generation of teachers and professionals working with learners who use AAC systems have not received any training in reading and writing instruction for persons with severe disabilities. The majority (78%) of the teachers who responded to the survey by Light and colleagues (1992) reported that they had received no training in teaching reading and writing to students who use AAC. McDaniel and DiBella-McCarthy (1989) suggest that teachers are most successful when they are knowledgeable and confident in their own teaching abilities and methods. Opportunities for inservice training are required to provide information on instructional theory and techniques to teachers working with students who use AAC. University programs for teacher education should be encouraged to provide preservice training for special educators in literacy instruction for students with severe disabilities.

Integrating literacy instruction with other activities

With better education, parents and educators are more apt to develop positive and realistic expectations for literacy learning for students who use AAC. These expectations must be translated into time, increased motivation, and appropriate activities in order to ensure successful outcomes. The priorities set by parents and teachers will no doubt have an impact on the time and motivation given to formal instruction and informal learning opportunities. Since reading and writing are not considered to be top priority by most parents of these children, such activities may receive less attention than other activities considered to be of greater importance. Within the home environment, the heavy demands of daily caregiving routines may leave little time or energy for literacy-related activities. Within school programs, therapy activities and caregiving demands may consume major portions of the day with little time left for reading and writing instruction. Koppenhaver and Yoder (1992) reviewed the literature on educational programs for students with severe speech and physical disabilities and concluded that these students receive significantly less instructional time within the school day than their nondisabled peers. As one of the teachers participating in the study by Light and colleagues (1992) noted, "All of the therapists are competing for time—power chair driving, toilet training, etc., etc." Obviously, the time for instruction is limited, and the need for intervention is great in many areas.

Parents and professionals may frequently be overwhelmed by the feeling that there is "so little time and so much to do." One solution to this dilemma is to integrate literacy instruction with other activities in the student's educational program and home routine (Blackstone, 1989). In order to maximize instructional time and effectiveness, reading and writing skills should be taught as part of larger skill clusters. For example, skill development in reading, writing, communication, and recreation might all be addressed within story reading activities with preschoolers who use AAC systems. Reading and writing vocabulary for shopping or eating out might be reviewed in the context of learning self-help or community social skills. A current focus of adult literacy programs for nondisabled adults is functional literacy instruction in which reading skills are developed in the context of learning necessary job skills (Strumf, 1991). Best practices suggest that skills should be taught systematically throughout the day, rather than in a single short instructional period (Calculator & Jorgensen, 1991).

Fostering collaboration between home and school

If literacy learning is to extend beyond formal instruction in the classroom, there needs to be close collaboration between home and school (Bodner-Johnson, 1986; Goldenberg, 1984). Light and Kelford Smith (in press) asked the parents in their study to indicate who should be responsible for teaching their children to read and write. Parents of preschoolers using AAC systems reported that the responsibility should be shared between teachers and mothers. These findings provide support for a collaborative model of literacy intervention with home and school working together. In many cases, communication between parents and teachers may be limited as evidenced by the lack of agreement between parent and teacher expectations and priorities reported by Light and associates (1992). There is a need for greater communication and collaboration between home and school to facilitate literacy learning by students using AAC systems.

Valuing writing skills

In reviewing parent and teacher priorities for students using AAC systems, it is of interest to note that both parents and teachers gave greater priority to reading skills than to writing skills (Light & Kelford Smith, in press; Light et al. 1992). This asymmetry is of particular note because the decreased emphasis on writing may result in a neglect of skill development in this area. Poor writing skills may restrict educational and vocational options. Kelford Smith and associates (1989) noted that "writing is the most widely used vehicle for the formal transmission of ideas and the most common medium of educational assessment" (p. 115). Writing skills may play a critical role in determining vocational opportunities for persons with severe physical disabilities who may have limited functional use of their hands. While there is assistive technology that offers access to text for those who cannot read (e.g., text readers), individuals who lack the literacy skills to compose written text have few options that will allow them to communicate effectively through print. Written communication skills offer persons who use AAC a means to enhance their communication skills and to bypass some of the limitations confronted in face-to-face interactions. When writing is neglected, the opportunity for students to benefit from the interrelationships of reading and writing activities is lost (Koppenhaver et al., 1991).

Developing effective instructional techniques

As indicated earlier, fostering positive and appropriate expectations and priorities for literacy development are first steps in the intervention process. In order to ensure functional literacy outcomes, however, these expectations must be followed by both formal and informal learning activities that are appropriately adapted to the needs of the learner. The research into literacy and AAC is still limited; we have much to learn about effective instruction to ensure that a greater number of students who use AAC are successful in learning to read and write.

•   •   •

The research available on expectations and priorities for literacy learning with children using AAC is limited. The studies to date are descriptive and rely exclusively on parent and teacher report. Ongoing research is required to extend our empirically based knowledge of literacy and AAC. Four main research questions with regard to expectations and priorities need to be investigated.

First, professionals need to develop a better understanding of the expectations and priorities held by parents, teachers, other professionals, and consumers who use AAC. Second, the role these expectations and priorities play in determining literacy outcomes must be investigated. What impact do parent, teacher, and student expectations have on behavior day to day? What impact do they have on final outcomes? Longitudinal studies are required to investigate the process of literacy learning and the factors that facilitate this development at different points in a student's development. Third, research on how expectations are formed and how they can be modified is needed. What factors contribute to the formation of positive expectations by parents, educators, and students? What impact do parent and professional education and information dissemination have on expectations for literacy acquisition and ultimately on literacy attainment? Finally, research is needed to develop better maps of literacy learning for students using AAC systems. Appropriate assessment procedures must be developed to assist in identifying students' current skill levels and in evaluating the impact of instructional procedures. Longitudinal research is required to identify appropriate expectations for future literacy development and to determine effective instructional techniques. Current knowledge about expectations and priorities should be used to develop more effective intervention programs. As new knowledge is applied, educators, professionals, parents, and consumers need to share their experiences with others in carefully documented case studies so that we can benefit from each other's successes and failures and learn from models of successful literacy attainment.

REFERENCES

Blackstone, S.W. (1989, January). ACN's guidelines for teaching literacy skills. *Augmentative Communication News*, p. 3.

Bodner-Johnson, B. (1986). The family environment and achievement of deaf students: A discriminant analysis. *Exceptional Children, 52,* 443–449.

Brattesani, K.A., Weinstein, R.S., & Marshall, H.H. (1984). Student perceptions of differential teacher treatment as moderators of teacher expectation effects. *Journal of Educational Psychology, 76,* 236–247.

Braun, C. (1976). Teacher expectation: Sociopsychological dynamics. *Review of Educational Research, 46,* 185–213.

Brown, C. (1954). *My left foot.* London, England: Secker and Warbug.

Calculator, S.N., & Jorgensen, C.M. (1991). Integrating AAC instruction into regular education settings: Expounding on best practices. *Augmentative and Alternative Communication, 7,* 204–214.

Cohen, S.G., McDonell, G., & Osborn, B. (1989). Self-perception of "at risk" and high achieving readers: Beyond reading recovery achievement data. In S. McCormick & J. Zutell (Eds.), *Cognitive and social perspectives for literacy research and instruction. Thirty-eighth yearbook of the National Reading Conference.* Chicago, IL: The National Reading Conference, Inc.

Cooper, H.M. (1979). Pygmalion grows up: A model for teacher expectation communication and performance influence. *Review of Educational Research, 49,* 389–410.

Dunn, N.E. (1981). Children's achievement at school-age entry as a function of mothers' and fathers' teaching sets. *The Elementary School Journal, 81,* 245–253.

Durkin, D. (1984). Poor black children who are successful readers: An investigation. *Urban Education, 19,* 53–76.

Featherstone, H. (1980). *A difference in the family.* New York, NY: Penguin.

Goldenberg, C.N. (1984, October). *Low-income Hispanic parents' contributions to the reading achievement of their first-grade children.* Paper presented at the meeting of the Evaluation Network/Evaluation Research Society, San Francisco, CA. (ERIC Document Reproduction Service No. ED 264 081).

Good, T.L., & Brophy, J.E. (1984). *Looking in classrooms* (3rd ed.). New York, NY: Harper & Row.

Harris, D. (1982). Communicative interaction processes involving nonvocal physically handicapped children. *Topics in Language Disorders, 2*(2), 21–37.

Herriman, M. (1986). Metalinguistic awareness and the growth of literacy. In S. de Castell, A. Luke, & K. Egan (Eds.), *Literacy, society, and schooling.* Cambridge, England: Cambridge University Press.

Kelford Smith, A., Thurston, S., Light, J., Parnes, P., & O'Keefe, B. (1989). The form and use of written communication produced by physically disabled individuals using microcomputers. *Augmentative and Alternative Communication, 5,* 115–124.

Koppenhaver, D., & Yoder, D. (1990). *The literacy literature: Individuals with speech and physical impairments.* Paper presented at the Biennial Conference of the International Society for Augmentative and Alternative Communication, Stockholm, Sweden.

Koppenhaver, D., & Yoder, D. (1992). Literacy issues in persons with severe speech and physical impairments. In R. Gaylord-Ross (Ed.), *Issues and research in special education* (Vol. 2). (pp. 156–201). New York: Columbia University Teachers College Press.

Koppenhaver, D.A., Evans, D.A., & Yoder, D.E. (1991). Childhood reading and writing experiences of literate adults with severe speech and motor impairments. *Augmentative and Alternative Communication, 7,* 20–33.

Lee, J.M. (1985). *Teacher wait-time: Task performance of developmentally delayed and on-delayed young children.* Doctoral dissertation, University of Florida. Dissertation Abstracts International, 47, 04A.

Light, J., & Kelford Smith, A. (in press). The home literacy experiences of preschoolers who use augmentative communication systems and of their nondisabled peers. *Augmentative and Alternative Communication.*

Light, J., Koppenhaver, D., Lee, E., & Riffle, L. (1992). *The home and school literacy experiences of students who use AAC systems.* Manuscript in preparation.

Marriner, N., Yorkston, D., Dowden, P., & Dudgeon, B. (1989, November). *Mapping augmentative communication programs.* Miniseminar presented at the annual convention of the American Speech-Language-Hearing Association, St. Louis, MO.

McDaniel, E.A., & DiBella-McCarthy, H. (1989). Enhancing teacher efficacy in special education. *Teaching Exceptional Children, 21*(4), 33–38.

McNaughton, D. (1991). *An investigation of the spelling skills of nonspeaking physically disabled adults.* Unpublished manuscript, The Pennsylvania State University, Department of Special Education, University Park, PA.

McNaughton, D., & Tawney, J. (in press). Comparison of two spelling instruction techniques for adults who use augmentative and alternative communication. *Augmentative and Alternative Communication.*

Palardy, J. (1969). What teachers believe—what children achieve. *Elementary School Journal, 69,* 370–374.

Parsons, J.E., Adler, T.F., & Kaczala, C.M. (1982). Socialization of achievement attitudes and beliefs: Parental influences. *Child Development, 53,* 310–321.

Parsons, J.E., & Ruble, D.N. (1977). The development of achievement-related expectancies. *Child Development, 48,* 1,075–1,079.

Picou, S.J., & Carter, M.T. (1976). Significant other influence and aspirations. *Sociology of Education, 49,* 12–22.

Seginer, R. (1983). Parents' educational expectations and children's academic achievements: A literature review. *Merrill-Palmer Quarterly, 29,* 1–23.

Strumf, L. (1991, October). What makes this hard? Workplace literacy and functional context instruction. *Mosaic: Research Notes on Literacy,* pp. 1–6.

Thompson, T.S., Alexander, K.L., & Entwhistle, D.R. (1988). Household composition, parental expectations, and school achievement. *Social Forces, 67,* 424–451.

The head-injured student returns to school: Recognizing and treating deficits

Jean L. Blosser, EdD, CCC–SLP
*Associate Professor of Speech–Language
    Pathology
Director, Speech and Hearing Center
Department of Communicative
    Disorders
University of Akron
Akron, Ohio*

Roberta DePompei, MA, CCC–SLP
*Associate Professor of Speech–Language
    Pathology
Department of Communicative
    Disorders
University of Akron
Akron, Ohio*

DUE TO GREAT improvements in overall treatment during the rehabilitation process, a significant number of head-injured students return to the educational setting following physical recuperation. Because of the complexity of the school setting and demands placed upon students at all levels, the reentering head-injured student is likely to encounter difficulties due to cognitive–communicative, physical, behavioral, and emotional problems, or a combination of all (Savage & Carter, 1984).

Since learning is a language-based process (Berlin, Blank, & Rose, 1980; Silliman, 1984; Wiig & Semel, 1980), the student's success upon return to school will depend on the ability to communicate effectively with others and perform appropriately on academic tasks and in classroom situations. When a head injury occurs, there is often a breakdown of the language processes, which can result in disorientation, disorganization of verbal activities, stimu-

Top Lang Disord, 1989, 9(2), 67–77
© 1989 Aspen Publishers, Inc.

lus-bound responses, reduced capacity for learning, and reduced ability to process incoming information. Rosen and Gerring (1986) point out that difficulties with memory, judgment, pragmatic skills, and problem solving will cause the most significant readjustment problems for the head-injured student. These problems may be reflected in the student's expression and understanding of language within the context of the school setting. The head-injured student who attempts to return to school with deficits in these areas can be expected to experience some difficulties, especially with performance in academic subjects and relating to others. Such difficulties must be recognized and understood by teachers and clinicians who will be responsible for working with the student upon reentry. Teaching strategies that will enable the student to benefit maximally from the educational experience must be employed.

Several questions emerge concerning the impact of the head-injured student's cognitive–communicative deficits upon school performance and relationships with others within the school setting, and concerning the educator's response to these deficits:

- What makes the head-injured student different from students with other handicaps?
- How are the cognitive–communicative deficits that result from the injury reflected in the student's classroom behavior and academic performance?
- Which teaching strategies can be used to help the student achieve maximum potential in terms of the learning situation?

- Which resources can be employed to increase communication skills?
- Which teaching behaviors can be used while working with the head-injured?

The first question points to the need for educators to learn about head injury as distinct from other handicaps. Since consideration of this population's return to school is relatively recent, attention needs to be given to their uniquely different characteristics. The second, third, and fourth questions address the specific cognitive–communicative deficits of the head-injured, how they may be exhibited in the classroom, and how they may be modified. The fifth question concerns the strategy employed to assist the student to improve cognitive–communicative skills so that learning can reach its maximum potential.

THE EDUCATOR'S PERSPECTIVE REGARDING THE HEAD-INJURED STUDENT

Educators who have not encountered a head-injured student often have limited understanding of the behaviors exhibited or the problems that are likely to occur among this population. Every head injury is unique. As has been mentioned, the head-injured student may demonstrate any combination of communicative, cognitive, physical, perceptual, behavioral, social, or emotional impairments. While several other handicapping conditions also result in deficits in these areas, the combination of deficits found in head-injured students cannot be as easily categorized and defined as is the case with other handicaps: One cannot generalize that most students with head injuries will behave in a similar manner. Individual differences among head-injured students will require a specific orientation for each.

The extent and variety of behaviors that each returning student exhibits must be taken into consideration when planning a reentry into the school setting. Educators need to be sensitized to the fact that the returning student may exhibit a number of disabilities, ranging from severe to mild, in several skill areas. The disabilities may lack consistency, and it will be difficult for those planning for the student to make generalizations based on performance in any one area.

Educators must be aware of the differences between this group and other handicapped groups in order to plan appropriately for class placement and participation. The head-injured student is not a "peer" of other handicapped students. The head-injured student did not begin his or her academic career as a handicapped student; the learning and communication handicaps were acquired. Listed below are some characteristics of the head-injured that make them different from individuals with other disabilities (Rosen & Gerring, 1986; Ylvisaker, 1985; Blosser & DePompei, 1987; DePompei & Blosser, 1987). The head-injured student typically has

- a sense of being normal that persists from the premorbid period
- discrepancies in ability levels
- a previous history of successful experiences in academic and social settings
- inconsistent patterns of performance
- variability and fluctuation in the recovery process, resulting in unpredictable and unexpected spurts of recovery
- more extreme problems with generalizing, integrating, or structuring information
- poor judgment and loss of emotional control, which cause the student to appear to be emotionally disturbed at times
- cognitive deficits that, although present in other handicaps, are more uneven in extent of damage and rate of recovery
- combinations of handicapping conditions that do not fall into usual categories of disabilities
- inappropriate behaviors that may be more exaggerated than the behaviors of students with other handicaps (e.g., greater impulsivity or distractibility)
- a learning style that requires the use of a variety of compensatory and adaptive strategies
- some intact high-level skills (making it difficult to understand why the student will have problems in performing lower-level tasks)
- a previously learned base of information that facilitates rapid relearning.

COGNITIVE–COMMUNICATIVE DEFICITS, CLASSROOM BEHAVIORS, AND TEACHING STRATEGIES

Depending on the site and extent of the injury, any number and combination of cognitive–communicative deficits may occur. These impairments will be demonstrated through the syntactic, semantic, phonologic, metalinguistic, and/or pragmatic behaviors exhibited by the student. Some of the cognitive–communicative impairments that will most affect classroom performance are impaired attention, inefficient processing of information, inability to remember and/or recall information, poor judgment, disorganization, inability to concentrate, inability to complete executive functions, ineffective problem-solving skills, difficulty with processing abstract information, difficulty with learning new information or rules, and inappropriate social communication behaviors. Difficulty in these areas is often reflected in the student's expression and understanding of language. Communication may be characterized by language comprehension deficits, word-finding problems, reduced or inappropriate verbal output, and phonological errors, as well as by many other maladaptive behaviors.

The educator must develop an awareness of the student's cognitive–communicative strengths and weaknesses and respond to them in the classroom. Awareness can be developed by observing, analyzing, and interpreting the behaviors that the student exhibits during classroom activities and interactions. Delayed responses, inability to complete class assignments, and irregular compliance with the school routine may be indicative of the student's problems with processing information presented or handling school demands. Head-injured students may exhibit immature behavior in comparison with peers and make decisions that are potentially dangerous. They may fail to realize the social consequences of comments and actions and may not learn from peers' positive examples or negative reactions. Performance during classroom activities may be deceiving. Answers to the teacher's questions may initially appear to be correct; however, further examination may reveal that they are simplistic and concrete.

Daily concentration on the development of cognitive–communicative skills is essential for obtaining maximum progress. Teaching activities and behaviors must focus on improving the student's expressive and receptive language skills to permit better functioning in these important areas.

It is impossible to present an exhaustive and uniform list of deficits and classroom behaviors that can be applied to all head-injured students because of the influence of such variables as age, extent of injury, developmental level, and academic expectations at each grade. The table that concludes this article (see Appendix) illustrates (1) the various types of cognitive–communicative deficits that head-injured students might exhibit; (2) an example of a classroom behavior that would characterize each deficit; and (3) skills that the student will need to learn in order to improve or compensate for the deficit, along with teaching strategies that can facilitate this learning. Numbers appearing in the last column of the table refer to specific resources and materials, listed in the key below the table, that are appropriate for teaching targeted skills. It is hoped that the reader will use the appendical table as a frame of reference for understanding and working with the head-injured student, classroom teacher, and family in the school context.

TEACHER BEHAVIORS

It is helpful for educators to monitor their own communicative behavior when working with the head-injured student. DePompei and Blosser (1987, 1988) suggest several behaviors that can be incorporated into teaching and interaction with the head-injured. The educator will need to exercise judgment in order to determine those with which they are comfortable and those to which a student will most likely respond. The authors suggest accompanying verbal instructions with written instructions and vice versa; avoiding figurative language; using pauses to direct the student's attention and to allow time for processing; providing examples, pictures, and written cues to illustrate important information and concepts; repeating instructions; and redefining new words and terms. Teaching materials should be concrete, and realistic efforts should be made to maintain a structured organization and routine throughout the student's day and to alert him or her to anticipated changes.

The head-injured student can also be encouraged to use several strategies to increase the likelihood of more accurate performance in the learning situation (DePompei & Blosser, 1988). Not all of these strategies will prove to be appropriate for all students. Therefore, it is suggested that teachers and clinicians spend some time experimenting with each to see which strategies yield effective results and under what circumstances. The strategies are as follows:

- Encourage the student to *reread* directions more than once, exercising care to underline or note the important elements.
- Ask the student to *repeat instructions verbatim* before initiating an activity.
- Verify the student's comprehension of directions by requesting that they be written or *restated* in different words.
- Ask the student to *proofread* assignments carefully before submitting them, checking for completeness and accuracy.
- Ask for *verbalization of the correct versus incorrect* aspects of the work.
- Provide the student with opportunities to *repeat assignments* at another time to see if performance can be improved.
- Invite the student to *ask questions* to clarify statements made in class.

• • •

The head-injured population is still new to the educational setting. Since resulting deficits are varied, head-injured students cannot be treated as a homogeneous group but must instead be considered unique and treated individually. Cognitive–communicative handicaps will most likely interfere with successful performance in academic and social situations. Educators who are faced with planning for the reentry of and teaching of head-injured students must understand these deficits, their influence on students' behavior, and specific teaching strategies in order to help students to achieve their maximum potential within the educational setting.

REFERENCES

Berlin, L.J., Blank, M., & Rose, S.A. (1980). The language of instruction: The hidden complexities. *Topics in Language Disorders, 1*(1), 47–58.

Blosser, J.L., & DePompei, R. (1987, April). *Facilitating classroom success for the closed head injured student.* Paper presented to the Council for Exceptional Children, 65th Annual Convention, Chicago.

DePompei, R., & Blosser, J.L. (1987). Strategies for helping head injured children successfully return to school. *Language, Speech and Hearing Services in Schools, 18,* 292–300.

DePompei, R., & Blosser, J.L. (1988). *Let's organize today! A calendar of daily cognitive–commuication activites for the head injured.* Danville, IL: The Interstate Printers and Publishers.

Rosen, C.D., & Gerring, J.P. (1986). *Head trauma: Educational re-integration.* San Diego: College-Hill Press.

Savage, R.C., & Carter, R. (1984, November-December). Re-entry: The head injured student returns to school. *Cognitive Rehabilitation, 2*(6), 28–33.

Silliman, E.R. (1984). Interactional competencies in the instructional context: The role of teaching discourse in learning. In G.P. Wallach & K.G. Butler (Eds.), *Language learning disabilities in school age children* (pp. 288–317). Baltimore: Williams and Wilkins.

Wiig, E.H., & Semel, E.M. (1980). *Language assessment and intervention for the learning disabled.* Columbus, OH: Charles E. Merrill.

Ylvisaker, M. (Ed.). (1985). *Head injury rehabilitation: children and adolescents.* San Diego: College-Hill Press.

Appendix

Understanding and meeting the classroom needs of the head-injured student

Cognitive–communicative deficits	Sample classroom behaviors	Target skills and teaching strategies	Resources[a]
Demonstrated difference between communication in informal situations and formal situations such as the classroom.	Student answers teacher's questions at a surface level; when pressed to give reasons why or more detail, student is unable to provide more information.	*Providing adequate and substantial information* Direct the amount and type of information provided by the student. Encourage conversations to develop by giving instructions such as "Tell me more," "How many did you see?"	1, 6, 9, 25
Length of sentences and use of gestures may be normal; depth of communication is not.	While student appears to do quite well conversationally during social situations, classroom speaking lacks detail and depth.	Role play formal conversations in small groups. Direct the context of the student's responses with your own verbal models, cues, and leading questions.	
Communication is tangential (rambling).	Student's conversations tend to ramble, with no acknowledgment of the listener's interest or attention.	*Topic maintenance* When the student begins to deviate from the topic, either provide a nonverbal cue or stop student from continuing.	13, 14
	Conversations may be topic-related but not exactly what is desired or germane to the discussion (e.g., when asked to name the major food groups, the student might begin a discussion about irrigation and growing crops).	Teach the student to recognize nonverbal behaviors indicating lack of interest or desire to make a comment. (Work on this skill during private conversations with the student.) Teach beginning, middle, and end of stories. Stop the student's response and restate the original question, thus focusing the student's attention on the key issue.	
Word retrieval errors	Student's answers contain a high proportion of "this," "that," "those things," "whatchamacallits," etc.	*Word recall* Teach the student association skills and give definitions of words that he or she cannot recall.	15, 31

Cognitive–communicative deficits	Sample classroom behaviors	Target skills and teaching strategies	Resources°
Verbal reasoning ability is reduced.	Student has difficulty providing answers on fill-in-the-blank tests.	Teach memory strategies (rehearsal, association, visualization, etc.).	5, 6, 10, 11, 31
	In algebra class, the student may arrive at a correct answer but not be able to recite the steps followed to solve the problem.	*Problem solving* Teach inductive and deductive reasoning at appropriate age levels. *Reasoning* Privately (not during classroom situations or in front of peers), ask the student to explain answers and provide reasons.	
Reduced ability to use abstractions in conversation (ambiguity, satire, inferences, drawing conclusions)	Student says things that classmates interpret as satirical, funny, or bizarre, although they were not so intended.	*Semantics* Teach the student common phrases used for satire, idioms, puns, etc.	5, 8, 13, 14
Delayed responses	When called upon to give an answer, the student will not answer immediately, appearing not to know the answer.	*Processing* Allow extra time for the student to discuss and explain. Avoid asking too many questions.	
Inability to describe events in appropriate detail and sequence	When student relates an experience, details are out of order, confused, or overlapping. Student cannot explain to another student the directions for playing a game in physical education class.	*Sequencing* Teach sequencing skills. Direct the context of the student's responses.	2, 3, 4, 5, 6, 12, 17, 18, 21, 22
Inadequate labeling or vocabulary to convey clear message	Student inappropriately labels tools in industrial arts class	*Semantics* Teach the student vocabulary associated with specific areas and classroom activities.	1, 6, 7, 9, 13, 17, 18, 23, 26, 31

Deficit	Example	Strategy	References
Inability to determine the salient features of Wh-questions asked, information communicated, or assignments read	Student completes the wrong assignment (e.g., Teacher requested that the class complete problems 9–12; this student completes problems 1–12.).	*Organization* Encourage the student to write assignments in daily log.	17, 18, 24, 29, 31
Inability to determine the specific aspects of questions that need to be answered	When answering questions about the details of a history lesson, student gets the details confused. When asked specific questions, student's responses may be related but not exact. Student is unable to decipher long story problems.	*Finding the facts* Ask questions that will elicit the student's recall of important facts.	
Inability to organize information mentally, whether presented verbally or in written form	Student performs steps of a science project out of sequence, either fixating on one step or performing the most apparent step ("I knew the other steps, I just didn't need to do them.")	*Sequencing* Provide the student with written 3- and 4-step sequences to sort and organize. Do not allow the student to skip steps in a demonstration, even if he or she claims to know what to do.	4, 5, 10, 11, 15, 16
Inability to analyze and integrate information received	Student executes written directions in an unorganized and incomplete manner. Student goes to the gymnasium for a program when it was announced that it would be held in the auditorium.	*Direction following* Directions should be written in numbered steps rather than in paragraph form.	16, 19, 20
Tendency to be easily overloaded by high amounts of oral information presented during classroom instruction	Student appears to be daydreaming and nonresponsive while the teacher is lecturing or giving instructions	*Focusing attention* Use pauses when giving classroom instructions to allow for processing information. Use short, simple sentences when explaining information.	
Inability to read nonverbal cues of others	Student seems to be unaware that the teacher or other classmates do not want to be bothered while they are working.	*Social awareness* Use preestablished nonverbal cues to alert the student that behavior is inappropriate. Explain what was wrong with the behavior and what would have been appropriate.	27, 28, 30

Cognitive–communicative deficits	Sample classroom behaviors	Target skills and teaching strategies	Resources°
Difficulty comprehending spoken messages if presented in complex terms, rapidly, or at length	Student exhibits poor notetaking skills, unable to maintain the ability to sort out and note the important parts of the teacher's discussion.	*Comprehension* Use short, simple sentences; emphasize key points by voice variations, intonations, etc. Alert the student to the important topic being discussed.	1, 7, 9, 13
Difficulty understanding or recognizing a sequence of events	Even after being back to school for a while, student still gets lost in the daily routine of the school day (e.g., forgets that spelling follows math).	*Organization* Provide the student with a written schedule of daily school routine and a map of the rooms to be found.	
Difficulty maintaining attention, comprehension, and concentration	Student loses place while reading; is unable to relate information recently read; is easily distracted during reading assignments; is unable to complete silent reading and seatwork assignments at the same rate as classmates.	*Processing* Provide student with additional time to complete classroom and homework tasks. *Attention concentration* Because the student will most likely be processing at the best rate possible, provide with ample time for reading assignments. Reduce the amount of work to be read. Use summaries.	
Reduced ability to understand abstractness in others' language (ambiguity, satire, inferences, drawing conclusions, etc.)	Student misunderstands instructions and comments made; while classmates are responding to satire, jokes, a pun, etc., the student appears to be unaware of the source of humor.	*Semantics* Do not use these styles when presenting important information while teaching or trying to correct the student's behavior. Teach the student the meaning of idioms, figurative language, ambiguous phrases, etc.	5, 13, 14

*Key: Resources to supplement classroom materials

1. Bender, M., & Valletutti, P. (1982). *Teaching functional academics: A curriculum guide for adolescents and adults with learning problems.* University Park Press. 300 North Charles St., Baltimore, MD 21201.

2. Blosser, J. (1984). *Let's talk about it: A calendar of daily activities for teaching language skills at home (ages 4–8).* The Interstate Printers and Publishers, Inc., Danville, IL 61832.

3. Blosser, J., & DePompei, R. (1985). *Let's listen today: A calendar of daily events for teaching listening skills at home (ages 4–8).* The Interstate Printers and Publishers, Inc., Danville, IL 61832.

4. DePompei, R., & Blosser, J. (1988). *Let's organize today: A calendar of daily cognitive-communication activities for the head injured.* The Interstate Printers and Publishers, Inc., Danville, IL 61832.

5. Brubacker, S. (1983). *Workbook for reasoning skills.* Wayne State University Press, Detroit, MI 48202.

6. Carter, L., Caruso, M., Languirand, M., & Berard, M. A. *The thinking skills workbook: A cognitive skills remediation manual for adults.* Charles C. Thomas, Publisher, 2600 S. First Street, Springfield, IL 62717.

7. Craine, J., & Gudeman, H. (1981). *The rehabilitation of brain functions.* Charles C. Thomas, Publisher.

8. Greatsinger, C., & Waelder, P. (1978). *Practice in survival reading* (series of 7 books). New Readers Press, Publishing Division of Laubach Literacy International, Box 131, Syracuse, NY 13210.

9. Gruenewald, L. J., & Pollak, S. A. (1984). *Language interaction in teaching and learning.* University Park Press.

10. Harnadale, A. (1976). *Critical thinking: Book one.* Midwest Publications Co, P.O. Box 448, Pacific Grove, CA 93950.

11. Jaffe, C., & Roberts, B. (1984). *Thinkathon I.* Educational Impressions, Inc., Hawthorne, NJ 07507.

12. Kahn, C., & Hanna, J. (1983). *Working makes sense* (practical arithmetic series, 2nd ed.). Fearon Pitman Publishers, 6 Davis Drive, Belmont, CA 94002.

13. Kilpatrick, K. (1979). *Therapy guide for the adult with language and speech disorders. Volume I: A selection of stimulus materials.* Visiting Nurse Service, 1200 McArthur Drive, Akron, OH 44320.

14. Kilpatrick, K. (1981). *Therapy guide for the adult with language and speech disorders. Volume 2: Advanced stimulus materials.* Visiting Nurse Service, Akron.

15. Kilpatrick, K. (1983). *Working with words: Volume 3.* Visiting Nurse Service, Akron.

16. Kilpatrick, K. (1985). *Putting the pieces together: Volume 4.* Visiting Nurse Service, Akron.

17. Lazzari, A., & Peters, P. M. (1980). *HELP: Handbook of exercises for language processing. Volume I: Auditory discrimination, auditory reception, auditory association, auditory memory.* Lingui-Systems, Inc., 1630 Fifth Avenue, Moline, IL 61265.

18. Lazzari, A., & Peters, A. M. (1980). *HELP: Handbook of exercises for language processing. Volume II: Specific word finding, categorization, wh-questions, grammar.* Lingui-Systems, Inc.

19. *Mind benders.* Midwest Publications Co, P.O. Box 448, Pacific Grove, CA 93980.

20. Nash, G., & Nash, B. *Pundles.* The Stone Song Press, 51 Madison Avenue, New York, NY 10010.

21. Parsons, J. (1979). *Math a riddle I* (subtraction). Fearon Pitman Publishers.

22. Parsons, J. (1979). *Math a riddle II* (multiplication). Fearon Pitman Publishers.

23. Pelton, V. (1980). *Learning to live on our own* (series of 6 books: housing, communication, money, health & family living, it's the law, transportation, and government services). Professional Educational Services, P.O. Box 246, Cortland, OH 44410.

24. Rockowitz, M. *High school equivalency examination.* Barron's Educational Series, 113 Crossways Park Drive, Woodbury, NY 11797.

25. Schwartz, L., & McKenley, N. (1984). *Daily communication: Strategies for the language disordered adolescent.* Thinking Publications, 7021 West Lower Creek Road, Eau Claire, WI 54701.

26. Waelder, P. K. Caution: Fine print ahead. New Readers Press. Publishing Division of Laubach Literacy International, Box 131, Syracuse, NY 13210.

27. Wiig, E. *Let's talk: Dating.* Charles E. Merrill Publishing Co. A Bell and Howell Co., Columbus, OH 43216.

28. Wiig, E. *Let's talk: Making dates.* Merrill Publishing.

29. Wiig, E. *Let's talk: Asking for favors.* Merrill Publishing.

30. Wiig, E. *Let's talk: Sharing feelings.* Merrill Publishing.

31. Zachman, L., Jorgensen, C., Barrett, M., Huisingh, R., & Snedden, M. K. (1982). *Manual of exercises for expressive reasoning.* Lingui-Systems, Inc.

Index